AF664780

A PASSION FOR SNOWDROPS

A Passion for Snowdrops

A Personal Perspective

George G. Brownlee

Whittles Publishing

Published by
Whittles Publishing Ltd.,
Dunbeath,
Caithness, KW6 6EG,
Scotland, UK

www.whittlespublishing.com

Reprinted 2022

ISBN 978-184995-493-8

Printed in the UK by 4edge Ltd.

Chloe Rowan Meadowcroft

She encouraged me to write this book

Contents

Foreword

No flowers can offer assurance of brighter days in prospect like snowdrops. These little harbingers of the 'certain spring'[1] have enchanted us since the time of Classical Greece. Brownlee's veritable winter wonderland of a book is more than a gardeners' guide to snowdrops. This galanthophile's delight interweaves tips on snowdrop cultivation based on the author's 30 years' experience of growing snowdrops, with art, history and unique first-hand insights into galantamine – a drug derived from snowdrops for the treatment of Alzheimer's disease. It also delves headlong into a taxonomic tangle of snowdrops, explaining the botanical features that can be used to tease apart seemingly indistinguishable snowdrops from one another.

Brownlee is a passionate galanthophile who has grown over 100 different species and varieties of snowdrop in his garden in Oxford over the course of three decades. His own personal insights into snowdrop cultivation, and the problems faced by gardeners of snowdrops in the urban environment are prominent. Three garden-worthy varieties are recommended for beginners to start a collection and a further 15 for more experienced galanthophiles. A diary-style flowering sequence from October to April offers a novel approach to snowdrop cultivation that enables gardeners to select varieties that will flower over 6 months of the year.

Nomenclature features prominently in the book. An early English name 'Snowe Dropps' is revealed – a plant listed in 1615, in the garden of Richard Shanne of Yorkshire. This is nearly 20 years earlier than the previous earliest known reference to 'Snow drops' in the Johnson edition of Gerard's herbal of 1633. The origin of snowdrop woodcuts in European and English herbals published over 50 years apart is discussed; the reader will discover how some 3,000 woodcuts were shipped from the Antwerp publishers of Dodoens', Lobel's and Clusius' herbals to the London publishers in 1632 for Gerard's herbal of 1633, at a cost of 600 florins.

Another unique feature of the book is the chapter on 'snowdrop art'. Here, many historical snowdrop images are depicted from the earliest known, unambiguous snowdrop image in Dodoens' European herbal published in Antwerp in 1568, to more recent images from English herbals and floras. Advice from Jacquie Hibbert on how best to paint snowdrops also features. No other author on snowdrops has attempted such an extensive description of snowdrop art or has described the evolution of the different art forms depicting the flowers.

Finally, a snowdrop index offers brief descriptions of all the 133 snowdrops cited in the book, including the 22 recognised species, and over 100 different garden-worthy varieties, many of which are portrayed with stunning photography. This summary, which includes where and when the snowdrops were named, will certainly be of interest to the galanthophile.

A Glossary, Notes and Bibliography are provided for readers seeking further detailed information or references, as well as appendices to guide readers wishing to buy snowdrops or see them in cultivation. Of local interest, the author informs readers that the Oxford Botanic Garden – the UK's oldest botanic garden, founded in 1621 – has an excellent collection of snowdrops, as has the Oxford colleges: Worcester College and St Edmund Hall. Besides the UK, Brownlee includes references to collections in Ireland, The Netherlands, Germany, Belgium, the USA, Canada, Australia and New Zealand. This book is sure to engage the amateur enthusiast and the experienced galanthophile alike. We wish it all the success and appreciation it deserves.

Dr Chris Thorogood, Deputy Director and Head of Science, Oxford Botanic Garden and Arboretum

Professor Simon Hiscock, Director, Oxford Botanic Garden and Arboretum

Preface

'The first of these bulbous Violets riseth out of the ground, with two small leaves flat and crested, of an overworne greene colour, betweene the which riseth up a small and tender stalke of two hands high; at the top whereof commeth forth of a skinny hood a small white floure of the bignesse of a Violet, compact of six leaves, three bigger, and three lesser, tipped at the points with a light greene; the smaller are fashioned into the vulgar forme of a heart, and pretily edged about with greene; the other three leaves are longer, and sharpe pointed. The whole floure hangeth downe his head, by reason of the weake foot stalke wheron it groweth. The root is small, white and bulbous'.

'These plants do grow wilde in Italy and the places adjacent. Notwithstanding our London gardens have taken possession of most of them many yeares past'.

'Some call them also Snow drops'.

'Touching the faculties [medicinal properties] of these bulbous Violets we have nothing to say, seeing that nothing is set downe hereof by the ancient Writers, nor any thing observed by the moderne; only they are maintained and cherished in gardens for the beautie and rarenesse of the floures, and sweetnesse of their smell'.[2]

I first bought snowdrop bulbs over 30 years ago to grow in my own urban garden in Oxford. Their main attraction was that they flowered in winter when little else was visible. Their whiteness shone through the dark, damp winter months and was good for my well-being. Gradually, over the years, my collection of snowdrops grew, and I became a galanthophile growing over 100 different varieties in my garden.

I have written this book to pass on my knowledge for growing snowdrops to others, first by describing how to cultivate them and second by mentioning varieties to grow without spending a fortune.

But this book is more than a guide to growing snowdrops because it reflects my passion for these small, white, iconic plants. Thus, I include two chapters on the order, or *sequence,* of flowering of different snowdrop varieties in my own garden from early-flowering autumn snowdrops, e.g. Queen Olga's snowdrop or Peshmen's snowdrop, to those still flowering at the end of the season in early April in the UK. After meeting a botanical artist, Jacquie Hibbert, I wrote a chapter on 'snowdrop art' tracing the history of the various media used to illustrate snowdrops over the ages. I describe the evolution of published snowdrop images from the earliest known snowdrop 'woodcut', which appeared in Dodoens' herbal published in Antwerp in 1568, through to artists illustrating snowdrops from the seventeenth to twentieth centuries. This chapter ends with advice from Jacquie as how best to paint snowdrops. My interest in the history of snowdrops extends to when, and by whom, individual cultivars were named, to which varieties are virus-infected, and the medicinal use of the drug 'galantamine' present in snowdrops.

An unexpected, and unintended, consequence of government's stay-at-home or 'lockdown policy' during the coronavirus pandemic of 2020 – where going to work is discouraged to avoid infecting others – is that people have more time to spare for hobbies. It is no surprise that gardening has enjoyed a remarkable resurgence – even among people living in flats with no garden, other than a balcony or windowsill to enjoy their plants. As Monty Don said, 'We don't look after the garden, the garden looks after us.'

Cultivation of snowdrops should benefit the well-being of anyone who might suffer under any government's lockdown policy. My own demeanour improved when I noticed the autumn-flowering Queen Olga's snowdrops emerging in early October 2020 in my own garden.

This encouraged me to get out and enjoy the garden when the daylight hours were drawing in.

This book makes no attempt to compete with more specialist snowdrop books, in which many hundreds to thousands of snowdrop varieties are described.[3] I recommend these books if further botanical or historical information is needed beyond the scope of my book.

Acknowledgements

I was encouraged to write this book by my wife, Susan. My granddaughter, Chloe Meadowcroft, enthusiastically helped me in the initial stages of writing, suggesting I should avoid Latin names of plants, where possible – advice I took on board.

Many people, too numerous to mention, have encouraged me in my passion for growing snowdrops. Early on, I was stimulated to grow different varieties of snowdrops by viewing the extensive collection at Foxgrove Plants, Berkshire, and at Colesbourne Park, Gloucestershire. More recently, Susan Kasper, head gardener at St Edmund Hall, Oxford, encouraged me to expand my collection, as has Simon Bagnall, head of gardens and grounds at Worcester College, Oxford. Both colleges have extensive displays of their own snowdrops and are open to the public. I am grateful to Susan Kasper for correcting errors in a late draft.

I thank Jacquie Hibbert, in particular, for inspiring me to write a chapter on 'snowdrop art' and for her advice on painting snowdrops. Professor Simon Hiscock, Director, Oxford Botanic Garden and Harcourt Arboretum, and Dr Chris Thorogood, Deputy Director and Head of Science, gave invaluable help on my draft manuscript and contributed to this book by writing a Foreword. They, like me, are passionate about snowdrops.

Simon Biddulph of Rodmarton Manor, Gloucestershire, helped me in my entry (in 'Famous galanthophiles') for his late mother, Mary Biddulph, who was a galanthophile at Rodmarton Manor, Gloucestershire, in the 1960s–1970s. He also gave me details of when he introduced the cultivars 'Rodmarton Sirius', 'Rodmarton Regulus' and 'Rodmarton Capella' into circulation.

I thank Professor Henry R. Woudhuysen, Rector at Lincoln College, Oxford, and Dr Dirk Imhof, curator of book and archives, Museum Plantin-Moretus, Antwerp, for advice on the use and reuse of woodblocks in sixteenth and seventeenth century herbals.

Ms Anne Chesher and Dr Daryl Green of Magdalen College Library, Oxford, gave me unstinting help in accessing and copying images from their Goodyer Archive. Professor Stephen Harris, Druce curator, Sherardian Collection, Department of Plant Sciences, Oxford, introduced me to the *Hortus Floridus* of de Passe. Ms Sophie Wilcox kindly assisted me in accessing the snowdrop images. I thank the University of Oxford, Bodleian Library for permission to publish images from Dodoens, 1568 and from de Passe, 1614.

I thank the University of Eichstätt-Ingolstadt, Germany, for permission to publish Plate 361 from Besler's 1613 edition of the *Hortus Eystettensis*; and the Duke of Beaufort, Badminton, UK, for permission to publish part of Plate 16, showing a bunch of 'double' snowdrops from *The Duchess of Beaufort's Flowers* (1983). The State Hermitage Museum, St Petersburg, Russia, kindly allowed me to reproduce their photographic portrait of the Grand Princess Olga Konstantinovna, Russia (1867).

ONE

INTRODUCTION

Beautiful, pretty,
Snowdrops in the garden now
Water dropping off

Haiku by Chloe Meadowcroft (aged 9)

The aim of this book is to encourage everyone with a garden, however small, to grow snowdrops. They are easy to grow and come up year after year delighting us with their early show of pristine white flowers. By choosing a few different species, or varieties, you will find that snowdrops are surprisingly interesting as one learns to recognize and appreciate the subtle differences between them. They can flower from October until the end of March providing interest for around six months of the year. Moreover, any one variety is usually in flower for more than a month, unlike most other flowering plants in which the flower is more ephemeral. Snowdrops need minimal attention, are not fussy as to the type of soil or their situation in the garden, and usually bulk up well from a few plants into large attractive clumps.

Snowdrops have become fantastically popular in the last few years, although snowdrop enthusiasts have existed for many years, certainly from late Victorian times.[4] Galanthophiles – those who are addicted to *Galanthus*, the Latin for snowdrops – will pay huge prices for the latest fashionable snowdrop. Yellow-tinged snowdrops, or even orange-tinged ones, or those with very greenish flowers are much in demand now. Prices of over £1,000 have been paid at auction for just one bulb. Nevertheless, it is perfectly possible to become an enthusiastic collector without spending such astronomical sums. With time, the latest snowdrops drop out of fashion and become cheaper. But be warned, if you become a galanthophile, you might be tempted to buy the occasional bulb costing £20–£40.

HISTORY OF THE SNOWDROP

The common snowdrop (*Galanthus nivalis*) (Figure 1) is sometimes found growing 'wild' in woods or on the verges of country roads in Britain but is not now thought to be native.[5] The words 'Snow drops' were first published in 1633 in the second Johnson edition of Gerard's illustrated herbal, which includes a woodcut figure (Figure 2) clearly recognizable as the common snowdrop.[6] Gerard writes, *'These plants do grow wilde in Italy and the places adjacent. Notwithstanding our London gardens have taken possession of most of them many yeares past.'* Thus, it is not surprising that a variation of the name snowdrop, 'Snowe Dropps', is known to have been used in England some 20 years earlier than Gerard.[7] Surprisingly, the snowdrop illustrated in Gerard's herbal of 1633 is reproduced from an even earlier book by the famous Flemish herbalist, Dodoens, in 1568.[8] We can, therefore, be certain that the snowdrop was already well known on the continent in the sixteenth century. It is quite possible that snowdrops were introduced to Britain much earlier by monks travelling between Europe and Britain.[9]

A second, larger variety of snowdrop was also illustrated in the Johnson edition of Gerard's herbal in 1633. In another equally famous English herbal of 1629 by John Parkinson,[10] both the smaller and the larger variety of snowdrop were clearly described, but not illustrated. Gerard called this larger snowdrop 'The Byzantine early bulbous Violet', clearly recognizing it came from Constantinople – the old name for Istanbul in Turkey (Figure 3). We now recognize this more robust snowdrop as a separate species, the Crimean snowdrop, *Galanthus plicatus*. Again, this image in Gerard had been 'borrowed' from an earlier European herbal by L'Ecluse (Clusius) published in 1601.[11]

There was a lot of confusion in the naming of snowdrops, and indeed plants in general, until Linnaeus, in 1735, introduced the

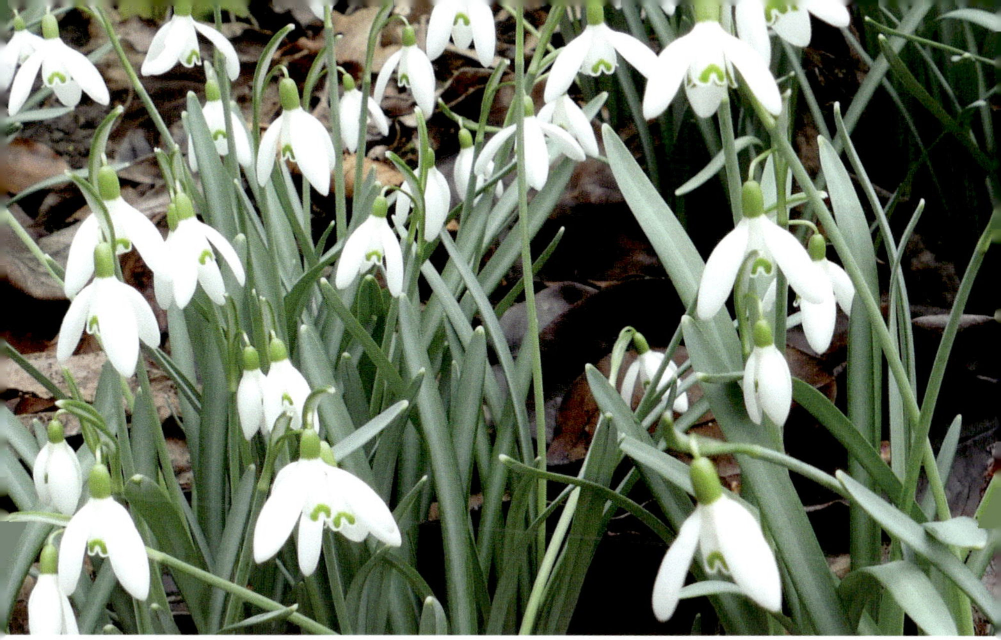

Figure 1 A clump of the common snowdrop, *G. nivalis*.

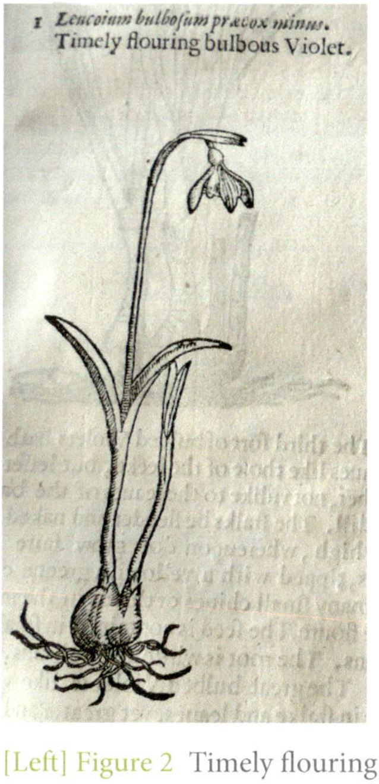

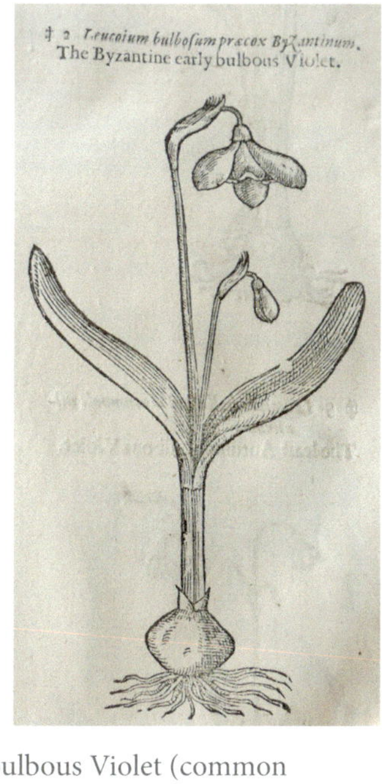

[Left] Figure 2 Timely flouring bulbous Violet (common snowdrop, *G. nivalis*) from Gerard, 1633.

[Right] Figure 3 The Byzantine early bulbous Violet (Crimean snowdrop, *G. plicatus*) from Gerard, 1633.

binomial system based on sexual characteristics. Snowdrops, in the sixteenth and seventeenth centuries, had been grouped together with snowflakes, now *Leucojum*, and had many different Latin, as well as English names. Three different English names – the 'white Bulbous Violet' or 'Narcissus Violet' or 'Theophrastus white Violet' – were in use in 1586.[12]

This reference to Theophrastus, who was a Greek herbalist of the fourth century BCE, suggests that the snowdrop (or the snowflake) was cultivated in Europe for over 2,000 years, although we cannot be certain of this because no images accompanying Theophrastus' writings have survived.[13]

A herb, today, is commonly a plant used to flavour food. But in the sixteenth and seventeenth century, a herbal was a collection of useful plants to treat various ailments afflicting the population. Herbals were the medical textbooks of that time, yet the snowdrop had no known healing properties. Nevertheless, snowdrops were included in these herbals, according to Gerard, because they were '*cherished in gardens for the beautie and rarenesse of the floures, and sweetnesse of their smell.*' Later botanists summed it up well and emphasized their early appearance in spring. Sowerby,[14] writing at the end of the eighteenth century, says, '*No plant is more generally cultivated, or more cordially welcomed as the herald of the approaching Spring.*'

WHAT IS A SNOWDROP LIKE, BOTANICALLY?

Snowdrops are classified within the amaryllis family (Amaryllidaceae), which includes many other familiar garden plants, such as daffodils, starflowers (*Ipheion*) and African lilies (*Agapanthus).* The most closely related plants to snowdrops are the snowflakes, *Leucojum.*[15]

The Latin name, *Galanthus* – after *gala,* the Greek for milk, and *anthos,* the Greek for flower – was introduced by Linnaeus for snowdrops. The name was inappropriate as snowdrops had never been associated with milk before. But with Linnaeus' authority, the name stuck.

The snowdrop is a bulb with two, or occasionally three, leaves arising directly from a bulb. There is a single flower stem, or occasionally two stems, with a single drooping flower with three outer petals (strictly tepals, or outer perianth segments) and three shorter inner petals (strictly

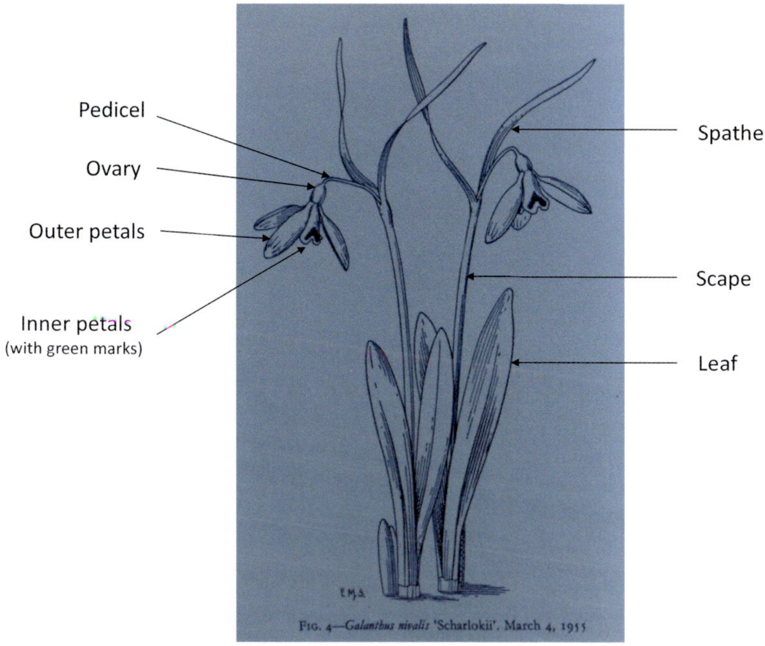

Figure 4 Visible parts of the snowdrop above ground.
(Adapted from Stern, 1956, p. 26).

inner perianth segments; Figure 4). All features of the snowdrop, e.g. leaves, scape (leafless stalk), spathe (modified leaves between the scape and pedicel, enclosing the flower in bud) and pedicel (flower stalk), are relevant in distinguishing different species and cultivars. However, the most important feature in species or cultivar identification is the flower, its size, its shape and particularly the markings on the inner petals. The three outer petals are generally white, although sometimes green-tipped, while the three inner petals usually have a small notch, or sinus, at their tip.

Figure 5 shows the variation in size and markings on the outside of the inner petals in 16 different varieties of snowdrops. These markings are a valuable, but not an absolute, aid to identification as they are not always a stable feature amongst different bulbs of the same variety. Note all 16 have a notched sinus. Some varieties have minimal green markings, e.g. 'Atkinsii', 'Brenda Troyle' and 'S. Arnott', whereas others

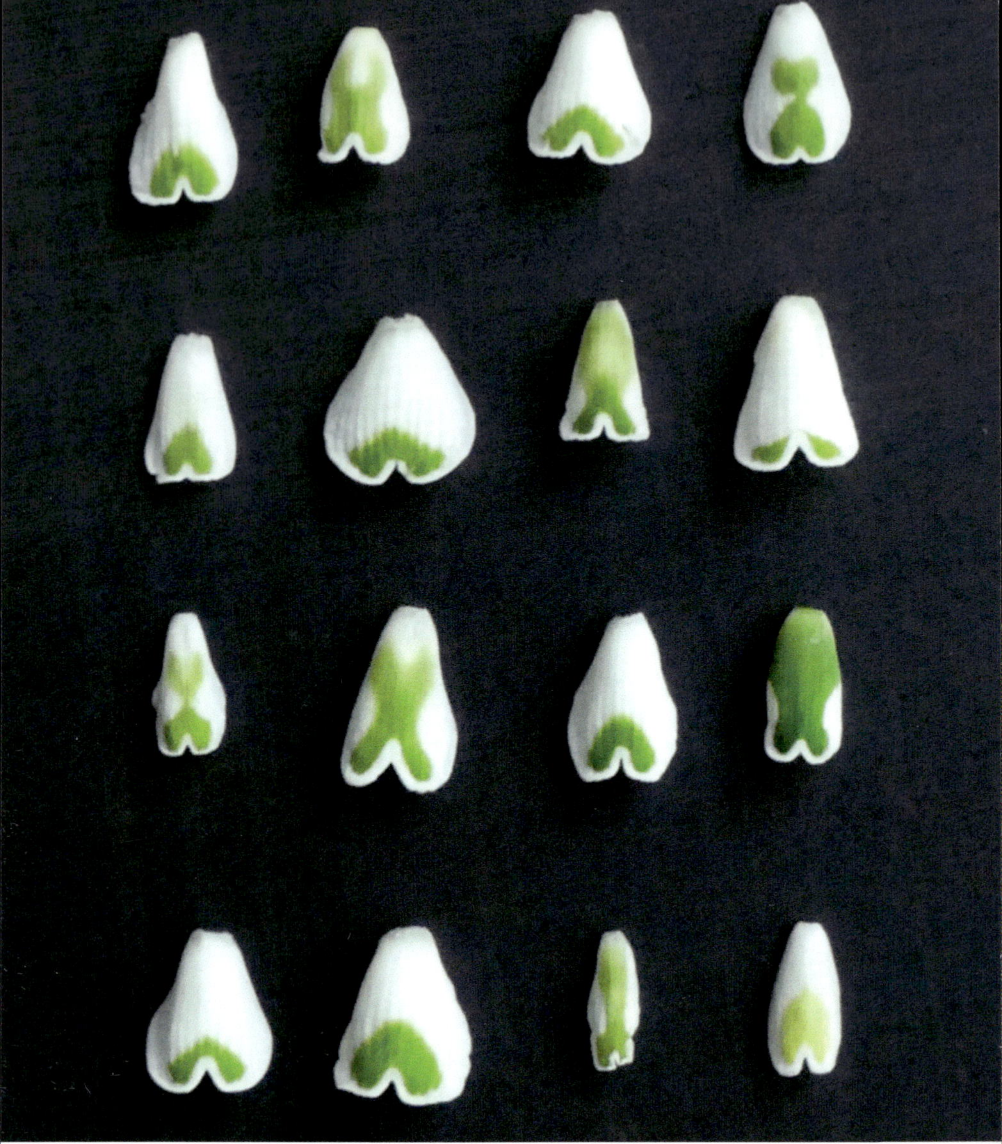

Figure 5 Markings on one inner petal, dissected from the flower of 16 different varieties of snowdrops showing the variation possible. The top of each petal lies adjacent to the ovary (not shown); the bottom, with the notched sinus, is unattached. The varieties, from top left to top right, are Row 1: 'Atkinsii', 'Augustus', 'Brenda Troyle', *G. elwesii*. Row 2: 'Galatea', *G. plicatus* ssp. *plicatus*, 'John Gray', 'Ketton'. Row 3: 'Kite', 'Little John', 'Magnet', 'Merlin'. Row 4: 'S. Arnott', 'Straffan', 'Wasp', 'Wendy's Gold'.

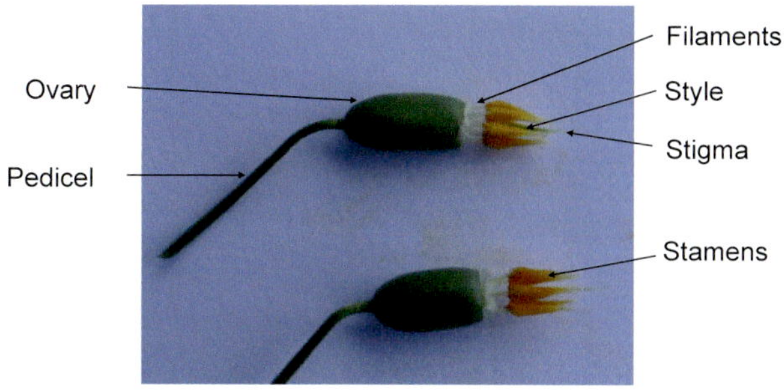

Figure 6 The stamens, filaments (structures joining the six stamens to the ovary), ovary and pedicel of two typical *Galanthus* flowers, with the six petals removed. The stamens and single style are visible, but the terminal stigma is too small to be seen clearly.

have an obvious green cross, e.g. 'Augustus', 'John Gray', 'Kite' and 'Little John'. Sometimes the petals are almost covered in green, e.g. 'Merlin', or have yellow instead of green markings, e.g. 'Wendy's Gold'.

Botanically,[16] we recognize the flowers have six stamens, an inferior ovary and a single style with its terminal stigma exceeding the length of the anthers (Figure 6). A ×10 lens is needed to see these features and other details clearly. The inside of the inner petals is also marked with green stripes, although these are not as distinct as those on the outside. After flowering and during seed formation, the leaves continue to lengthen and droop considerably. Some snowdrops flower

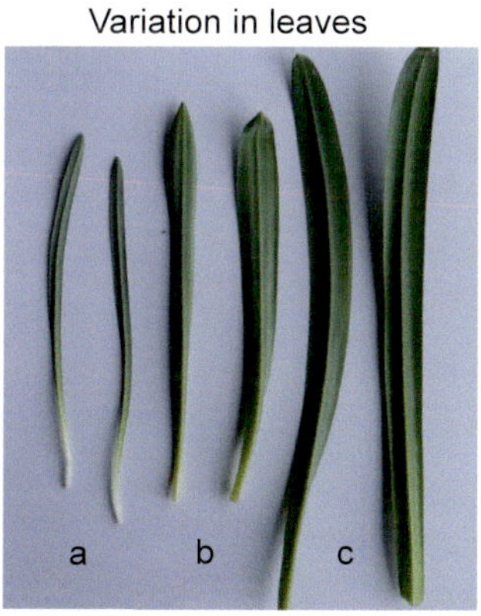

Figure 7 Back of leaves (in duplicate) of (a) the common snowdrop, *G. nivalis*, (b) Elwes' snowdrop, *G. elwesii* and (c) the Crimean snowdrop, *G. plicatus* ssp. *plicatus*.

in autumn with minimal leaves showing, but most flower in winter to early spring.

Snowdrop leaves vary in shape. Some are narrow, as in the common snowdrop (*G. nivalis*). Others are often wider, particularly in Elwes' snowdrop (*G. elwesii*) and in some Crimean (*G. plicatus*) cultivars. Leaf colour varies from shiny green – as in bluebell leaves – to light green and various shades of glaucous green. 'Glaucous' – a greyish or bluish-grey bloom covering the leaves – refers to the waxy finish on the leaves giving many snowdrop cultivars their attractive appearance. Figure 7 shows the variation in the back of the leaves of three varieties to emphasize the prominent midrib of the leaves, particularly in the Crimean snowdrop (*G. plicatus*). Some snowdrop varieties have leaves with distinctive ovoid (oval in outline) shapes, e.g. 'Augustus'. Others have a whitish midrib, e.g. Peshmen's snowdrop (*G. peshmenii*) and Queen Olga's snowdrop (*G. reginae-olgae*). Thus, the size, shape and colour of leaves can be an aid to identification in a collection of snowdrops.

22 DIFFERENT SNOWDROP SPECIES

Taxonomists now recognize 22 different snowdrop species, which are listed in Table 1 along with the date of their definitive naming as distinct species and their location in the wild. I have also suggested a common name for the more generally available species for those gardeners who dislike Latin names. For convenience, I classify species into those that are generally available from nurseries (common), those available from specialist nurseries (uncommon) and those that are more difficult to source (rare).

In the wild, snowdrops are found growing in Europe, Asia Minor and the Near East as far south as Sicily, Greece and Lebanon, and as far north as Germany and parts of Russia (Table 1). In the wild, the snowdrop is a woodland, often alpine species but some species, e.g. Peshmen's snowdrop (*G. peshmenii*), grow at sea level. However, many snowdrops have been introduced into countries all over the world and thrive successfully in a variety of habitats in the UK, Europe, the Americas, Australia, New Zealand and in Japan.

Snowdrop species are very difficult to tell apart even for the specialist because they have few distinguishing features. Detailed field work then

Table 1 Snowdrop species, their availability, when named, and their location in the wild

Species[a]	**Common**	**Uncommon**	**Rare**	**Common names**[b]	**When named**	**Location**[c] **(in the wild)**
G. elwesii	Yes			Elwes'	1875	Turkey, Balkans
G. nivalis	Yes			Common	1753	Europe, Caucasus
G. nivalis 'Flore Pleno'	Yes			Double	1703	
G. plicatus	Yes			Crimean	1819	Crimea, Turkey
G. woronowii	Yes			Woronow's	1935	Russia
G. alpinus		Yes		Alpine	1911	Caucasus, Turkey
G. gracilis		Yes		Slender	1891	Greece, Balkans, Turkey
G. peshmenii		Yes		Peshmen's	1994	Greece, Turkey
G. reginae-olgae		Yes		Queen Olga's	1876	Greece, Sicily
G. rizehensis		Yes		from Rize	1956	Turkey
G. angustifolius			Yes		1951	Russia
G. bursanus			Yes		2019	Turkey
G. cilicicus			Yes		1897	Turkey
G. fosteri			Yes		1889	Turkey, Syria
G. ikariae			Yes		1893	Greece
G. koenenianus			Yes		1994	Turkey
G. krasnovii			Yes		1963	Georgia, Turkey

Table 1 *Continued*

Species[a]	Common	Uncommon	Rare	Common names[b]	When named	Location[c] (in the wild)
G. lagodechianus			Yes		1947	Georgia, Russia
G. panjutinii			Yes		2012	Georgia, Russia
G. platyphyllus			Yes		1948	Georgia, Russia
G. samothracicus			Yes		2014	Greece
G. transcaucasicus			Yes		1909	Azerbaijan
G. trojanus			Yes		2001	Turkey

Notes: [a]Includes a double cultivar of *G. nivalis* 'Flore Pleno; [b]Suggested common names; [c]Locations are not exhaustive.

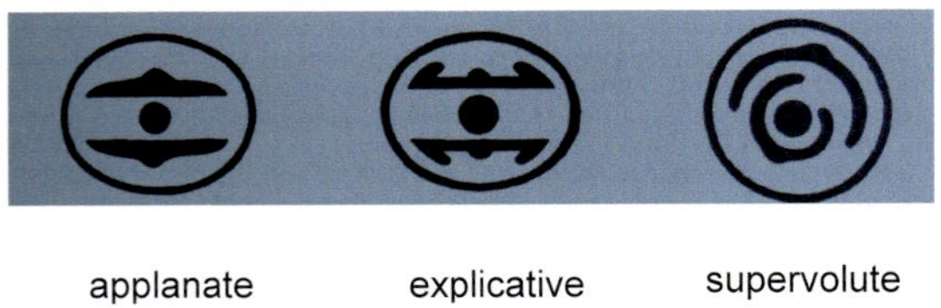

Figure 8 Diagram of types of snowdrop leaf vernation in cross-section. (Adapted from Stern, 1956, p. 26).

becomes important to establish whether a potential new snowdrop discovery is a novel species, as opposed to a naturally occurring variant or hybrid. Classification of snowdrops was highly problematic until Aaron Davis reclassified snowdrops in 1999,[17] although it is still possible that this classification could change in the future. The latest snowdrop to be classified as a new species, *G. bursanus*, was found in the Sea of Marmara region in northwest Turkey. It is autumn flowering and was described as recently as 2019.[18] Although only limited DNA sequencing has been used to lend weight to this classification, the 'phylogenetic tree' derived from limited DNA sequence of a few genes of snowdrops is consistent with the current number of species.[19] Subspecies – a plant with an established variation below the level of species – have been recognized in a few of the known snowdrop species.[20]

The taxonomy of snowdrops is based on quite subtle differences between snowdrops, which gardeners might not wish to study, although they can sometimes help resolve discrepancies in labelling of plants if varieties are muddled up.[21] Leaf vernation, or the appearance of the two leaves in bud, or where the leaves emerge from the soil, is one important taxonomic feature.

Applanate vernation describes where the two leaves lie flat against one another, as in the common snowdrop, *G. nivalis*, whereas explicative vernation describes the situation where leaves are bent back at their margins, as in the Crimean snowdrop, *G. plicatus*. Supervolute vernation is present when the two leaves are wrapped around one another, as in Woronow's snowdrop, *G. woronowii* (Figure 8). In practice, I find leaf vernation is mainly useful in the identification of the Crimean snowdrop because even the mature leaves have backward facing margins. Leaf colour, time of flowering and inner petal markings are other key distinguishing features used in defining species. The location of where plants are found in the wild (of little use to gardeners) is also used in distinguishing snowdrop species from one another.[22]

Hybrids and Cultivars

Many of the named snowdrops grown in gardens have long been thought to be hybrids, resulting from a cross between two different species. When hybridization occurs in nature the actual parental species may be suspected – from observing the new hybrid or from knowing where it was collected – but the parents will not be known for certain. Many of the named snowdrops are probably hybrids between the common snowdrop (*G. nivalis*) and the Crimean snowdrop (*G. plicatus*) or between Elwes' snowdrop (*G. elwesii*) and the Crimean snowdrop (*G. plicatus*).[23]

The opportunity for hybridization increases significantly when snowdrop species are grown together in gardens. Superimposed on this variation due to hybridization are seedlings with desirable properties that are noted by snowdrop enthusiasts and brought into cultivation. A good example of this is 'Diggory' – probably a *G. plicatus* seedling. These are caused by mutations in the ovum or sperm. Examples of other mutations are those giving rise to yellow ovaries and yellow markings on the flowers, or double ovaries, or green tips on the outer petals, or other forms of admired, even aberrant flowers. This explains why there are over 1,000 different named cultivars of snowdrops.

For some hybrids, however, the parental species are definitely known. The best known such hybrids were developed by Heyrick Greatorex, who crossed the double form of the common snowdrop (*G. nivalis* 'Flore Pleno'), with the Crimean snowdrop (*G. plicatus*) in the 1940–50s. These Greatorex doubles, which are more vigorous than the more diminutive parental double, were mainly named after Shakespearean characters. Although popular and widely grown, they are notoriously difficult to tell apart. The best of these doubles, according to Greatorex,[24] were 'Ophelia', 'Desdemona', 'Cordelia', 'Jaquenetta' and 'White Swan'. Personally, I think 'White Swan' is the best of the doubles, but 'Hippolyta' comes a close second.

ABBREVIATED NAMES FOR CULTIVARS

Many recognized and garden-worthy snowdrop cultivars are probably hybrids, or named varieties, often of unknown origin, as mentioned earlier. I find it is inconvenient to label my snowdrops – other than the species snowdrops – with their correct Latin species name, followed by the cultivar name. I simply use the cultivar name instead. In naming new cultivars, convention prohibits using a cultivar name if it had been used before. Therefore, the cultivar name is unique. For example, *Galanthus* 'Lady Beatrix Stanley' – an early double snowdrop, becomes 'Lady Beatrix Stanley'.[25]

TWO

GROWING SNOWDROPS IN YOUR GARDEN

BUYING

I prefer to buy snowdrops 'in the green'. Such plants – available from specialist nurseries in the snowdrop season – should have been recently dug out of the ground and are purchased by mail order usually in February or March. The advantage of buying in the green, over buying bulbs, is that you can judge where to plant them to fit in with other snowdrops or companion plants in your garden. The disadvantage – and this also applies to plants purchased growing in pots – is that there is inevitably some damage to the roots during transplantation. However, I have found that most snowdrops planted in the green flower the next year.

There are competing schools of thought as to whether it is better to purchase bulbs or to buy growing plants. Although it would seem to be advantageous to purchase snowdrops as bulbs in the autumn, the disadvantage of planting bulbs is the risk that they will be planted in the wrong place, for example unintentionally covering other bulbs already in place in the garden. I have also found that there are significant losses when planting bulbs, and the wrong snowdrop can emerge because of errors by the supplier including incorrect bulbs.[26]

PLANTING

Whichever way you buy snowdrops, they should be planted out in the garden as soon as possible in their permanent position. If this is not possible, plants purchased in the green must be unpacked and heeled in the ground without delay. This may not be possible if there has been a recent frost, in which case the plants must be kept in a frost-free place until they can be planted out. Snowdrops in pots must also be kept in a frost-free place until they can be transplanted as their roots are susceptible to frost damage.

Normally, plants should be planted at least three times deeper than the size of the bulb, if not deeper. Snowdrop bulbs can vary in size from the small common snowdrop (*G. nivalis*) bulb of 0.5–1 cm diameter, to larger bulbs like some cultivars of Elwes' snowdrop (*G. elwesii*) of 1–2 cm diameter, which are as large as daffodil bulbs. So it would be normal to plant the larger bulbs deeper than the smaller ones.

Plant in good, fertile, but not waterlogged soil, preferably in a group about 3 cm apart. I usually add grit to the soil to improve drainage, along with some compost. If planting in the green, attention should be paid to the depth of the previous planting and replant at a similar depth. It is important to water in after planting in the green to aid in the establishment of the plant, even if the soil is damp. Snowdrops will survive in most soils whether acid, neutral or alkaline, although extremely acid or alkaline conditions are reported to be unsuitable.

WHERE IN THE GARDEN SHOULD SNOWDROPS BE PLANTED?

This is very much up to individual preference and is obviously influenced by the size of your garden. Most snowdrops in the wild grow in deciduous woodlands. Few of us have a woodland garden to mimic these conditions, but nevertheless snowdrops can be grown very successfully in most gardens. It is often stated that they like some shade from deciduous trees or bushes to avoid the bulbs drying out in summer heat. Despite this advice, in Kew Gardens, London, snowdrops happily grow in their rockery area in full sun.

In practice, I have found that it is best not to be too concerned about the position of snowdrops in the garden – other than avoiding dense shade. For example, I would avoid planting too near a beech or privet hedge, or a large established tree, unless the soil is thoroughly worked by first digging in compost and grit.

Snowdrops take very little room, so are good plants for a small space and can usually be tucked in somewhere. It is a good idea to plant snowdrops where you can see them emerging in winter and early spring. But try planting in different positions in the garden, including a north-facing garden, to see which works out best. If you have a herbaceous border, they look great at the front or back of the border since the herbaceous plants will likely be dormant between January and April. Try to avoid growing in a mid-border position because the bulbs may be easily disturbed or dug up by mistake after their foliage has died down in late spring.

Snowdrops look good planted around deciduous shrubs or young fruit trees and the more vigorous cultivars grow quite happily in grass – especially if the grass is somewhat shaded in summer. To plant in grass, remove a spade-width of turf, fork the soil below the turf adding some gritty soil, then plant the snowdrops about 3 cm apart. After replacing the turf, breaking it up to accommodate the snowdrop foliage, firm in with your shoe or boot. The grass should not be mowed where snowdrops have flowered until the foliage has fully withered – usually by May.

DIVIDING

Most snowdrop cultivars are selected for good growth and normally grow well, producing offset bulbs each year. Do not disturb the bulbs after planting, just leave them to come up every year so they 'clump up' to produce an attractive display. It is unnecessary to cut off seed heads produced after flowering, as is often done with daffodils. Although clumps can be left for many years, they will eventually need dividing, with the possible exception of the common snowdrop.

How often clumps need dividing will vary and has to be decided by observation. Vigorous varieties, such as the Greatorex doubles, will go 'blind' (meaning they produce no flowers) if not divided after 5 years or so. However, I have never divided a few other slower growing varieties, e.g. 'Allenii',[27] which is a classic late snowdrop named in 1891 in honour of James Allen (Figure 9), or 'Anne of Geierstein',[28] which is another latish snowdrop, named around 1900 after the novel of the same name by Walter Scott (Figure 10).

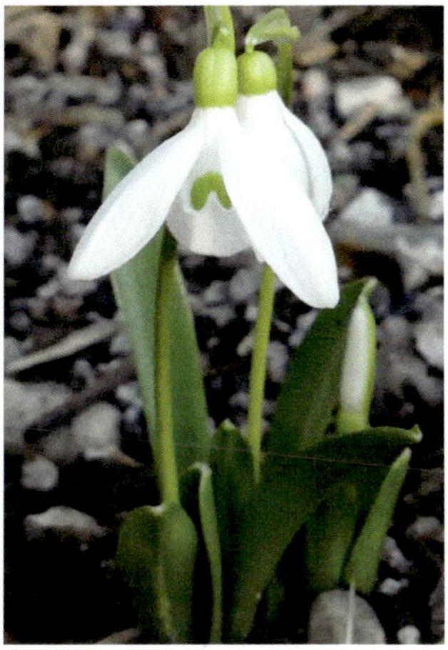

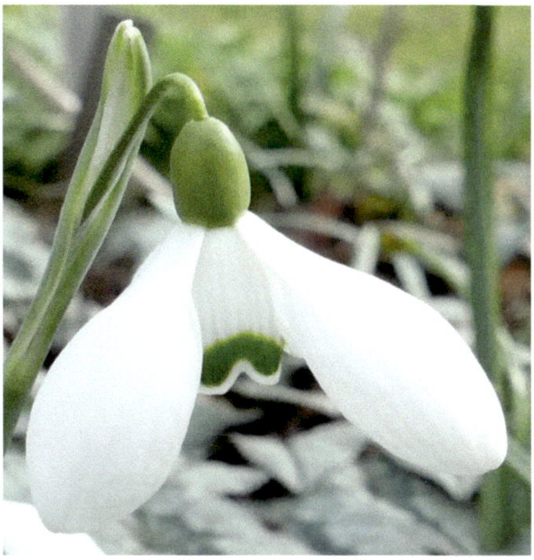

[Left] Figure 9 Allenii', a late, slow-growing classic snowdrop.

[Right] Figure 10 'Anne of Geierstein', another slow-growing classic snowdrop.

Clumps of snowdrops can be divided at any time during their growing period but are best divided in March or early April when their foliage is beginning to die back. Then there will be the least disturbance to their growth as long as transplantation is not delayed. Use a garden fork to dig up the snowdrop clump and then carefully tease apart the bulbs with the help of a hand fork to minimize disturbance to the roots. They can be planted elsewhere in the garden or simply, if space allows, be spaced about 3 cm apart in good fertile soil near the original plant. It is not necessary to tease apart every single bulb. When dividing, I often leave two to three bulbs together.

Commercially, specialist snowdrop growers use the technique of 'twin-scaling' to divide snowdrops, obtaining 20 or so bulbs from a single bulb. However, this technique[29] requires care, patience and the use of semi-sterile conditions, which the gardener may not want to bother with.

The growth of snowdrops in lawns is obviously affected by competition with the grass and they will clump up more slowly there. They will need dividing less often than snowdrops grown in garden soil. I grow two doubles in my lawn, the early double 'Lady Beatrix Stanley' and the taller double 'White Swan'.

LOOKING AFTER YOUR SNOWDROPS

Snowdrops need surprisingly little attention after planting. They are not killed by very hard frosts down to –20°C (Figure 11). Snowdrops can look most attractive after a snowfall, as is the case with 'Margaret Biddulph', with its prominent green markings, after a snowfall in early February (Figure 12).

However, some more specialist snowdrops, such as Peshmen's snowdrop (*G. peshmenii*) are less hardy.

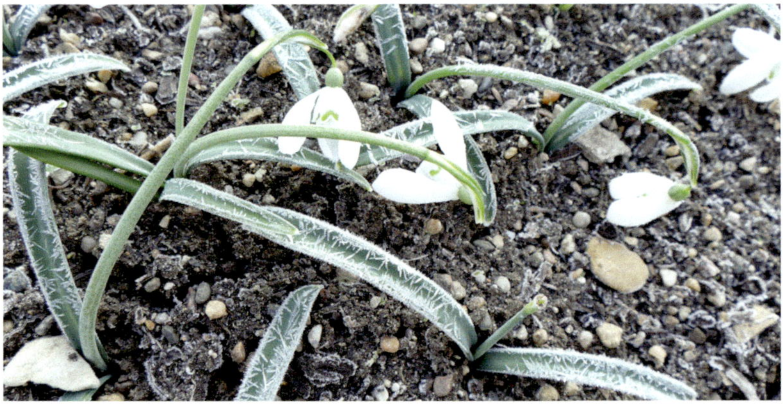

Figure 11 Hoar frost prostrating 'Hiemalis' in November.

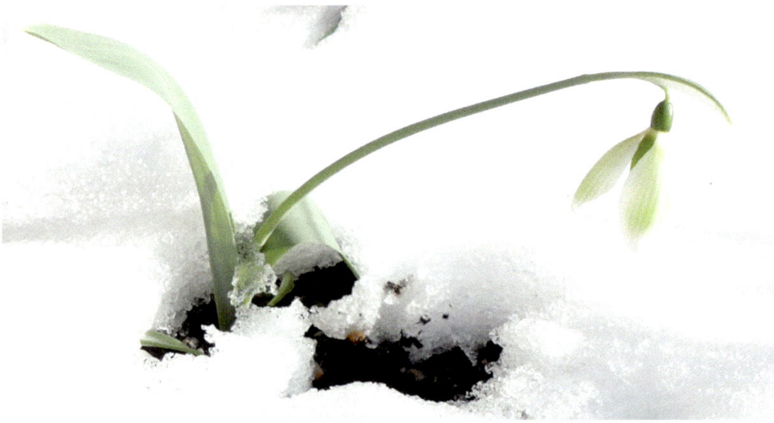

Figure 12 'Margaret Biddulph' emerging unscathed after a snowfall in early February.

Snowdrops do not need regular fertilizing with compost or other fertilizers. Some older books[30] positively warn against fertilizing them with manure, stating that 'nothing will kill them more quickly', although others recommend a top dressing with spent mushroom compost or an autumn feed of bone meal with some general fertilizer in the growing season.[31] I do not overfeed snowdrops but lightly top dress them with a mixture of soil, grit, a small amount of compost and sharp sand usually in autumn before the snowdrops emerge. Alternatively, if the snowdrops are growing where leaves accumulate in autumn, I recommend leaving the leaves to fertilize the snowdrops naturally.

Weeds or other plants can be a problem as they compete for space and soil nutrients. Snowdrops may fail to thrive because they are less vigorous. It is best to remove seedlings of primroses or Lenten rose (*Helleborus orientalis*) that are growing too close to snowdrops.

Look out for snowdrop seedlings. Most single snowdrops produce viable seeds, which will germinate to give new plants, potentially differing from their parent. Elwes' and Queen Olga's snowdrops have produced interesting variant snowdrops in my garden.

LABELLING

There is nothing more frustrating than getting snowdrop names muddled up. The problem is that many named varieties look very similar to one another. In some cases – the Greatorex hybrids – they may be almost impossible to tell apart.

All labelling of the position of snowdrops with labels inserted in the soil near the plant ultimately fails. My granddaughter, when she was 2 years old, proudly collected up all my snowdrop labels thinking I would be pleased. A head gardener of an Oxford College has resorted to hiding labels by burying them near the snowdrops, because the undergraduates enjoyed rearranging labels. Magpies and pigeons can peck and move labels at any time. The only permanent solution is to keep a record of the named snowdrop and a plan of the planting scheme, traditionally in a 'Garden Book', but often these days in a file on a laptop or other device.

Some gardeners dislike labels because they are unsightly, but I still like to label snowdrops, if only to remind me of the cultivar. White plastic labels are unsatisfactory as the labelling rarely survives more than one year. I prefer to label plants using pencilled aluminium labels firmly inserted in the soil. They retain their identification for about 10 years, but I still find one or two labels in my compost heap each year, because I have swept them up, by accident, when clearing leaves in the autumn.

DISEASES

According to Stern,[32] snowdrops are relatively free from pests and diseases. The reason for this, in part, is that snowdrops contain compounds which are toxic to most mammalian pests. A toxic compound, galantamine, which is present in snowdrops, snowflakes and daffodils, was isolated in the 1950s and presumably evolved to protect snowdrops from being eaten by predators. In fact, snowdrops are subject to diseases, especially fungal diseases. Gardeners should keep a watchful eye for any snowdrop that is not thriving in case it is diseased.

The most serious disease of snowdrops is from the fungus causing leaf scorch.[33] Treatment is problematic, and it is best to dig up and throw away infected bulbs. If the variety is valuable, bulbs can be treated with a fungicide and replanted elsewhere in the garden to see if the bulb survives, and then watching for any sign of infection. Other fungi, including *Botrytis,* attack shoots and leaves at ground level. The infected leaves or shoots are covered with a furry dense, grey mould. The slender snowdrop (*G. gracilis*) is prone to attack by this fungus. The rule is, whenever a snowdrop is not thriving, investigate by digging it up and preferably destroying it, thereby minimizing the chance of infecting other snowdrops.

Insects[34] can kill the bulb of a snowdrop by laying eggs in the bulb after accessing the bulb in late spring through the dying flower stem. Larvae hatch out and eat the bulb, presumably unaffected by toxins present in the bulb. The only evidence of disease is a failure of the plant to reappear the next year. All one can do is dig up and dispose of damaged bulbs. One precaution you can take is to block up the hole left by the dying stem of your snowdrop with some earth or sharp sand to stop further attack by these insects.

Viruses are known to be present in snowdrops, but the only virus to be positively identified is potato Y virus in 'Augustus', although this variety seems to grow happily despite the infection.[35] Other snowdrops that show yellowing and twisting of the leaves may also be virus-infected, such as 'Primrose Warburg' and 'Allenii', although I have seen no problems on my 'Allenii'. There is no treatment for virus infection other than to make sure the snowdrops are growing well. I have transplanted 'Primrose Warburg' after observing yellowing of the leaves and have noted some improvement in leaf colour after transplantation. Research[36] is needed to find out whether there is extensive, although not obvious, viral disease of snowdrops, because of the widespread occurrence of viruses in related plants, particularly daffodils.

Snails and slugs like to eat the flowers of snowdrops, attracted by the nectar (Figure 13). The early autumn-flowering Queen Olga's

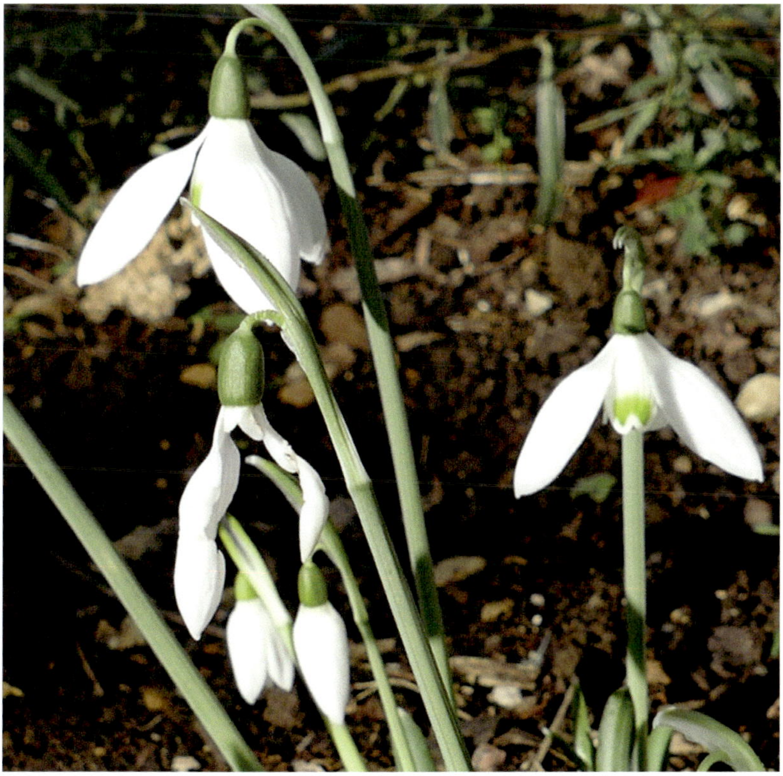

Figure 13 Slug or snail damage to the flower of Queen Olga's snowdrop (*G. reginae-olgae*) in October.

snowdrops and the late season snowdrops are particularly at risk because the warmer weather then encourages more snails and slugs to be active. Proprietary slug repellents can minimize damage.

Birds, mice and squirrels can disturb snowdrops, but the main problem is that their activity moves the plant labels around.

COMPANION PLANTS

Some gardeners like to plant companion plants that flower around the same time as snowdrops, as long as there is space for them. In early spring, the best companion plant is the red cyclamen (*Cyclamen coum*) or the yellow winter aconite (*Eranthis hyemalis*), or early-flowering daffodils. The contrast between the whiteness of the snowdrops and the red of *C. coum* is very pleasing to the eye (Figure 14). The dark purple Tommasini's crocus (*Crocus tommasinianus*) is also a good companion

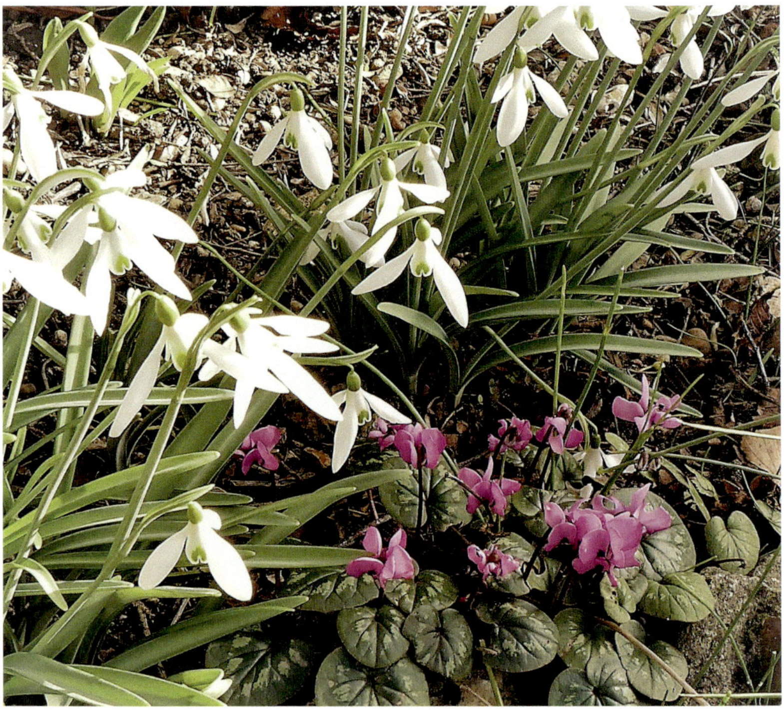

Figure 14 'James Backhouse' and *Cyclamen coum* in spring sunlight.

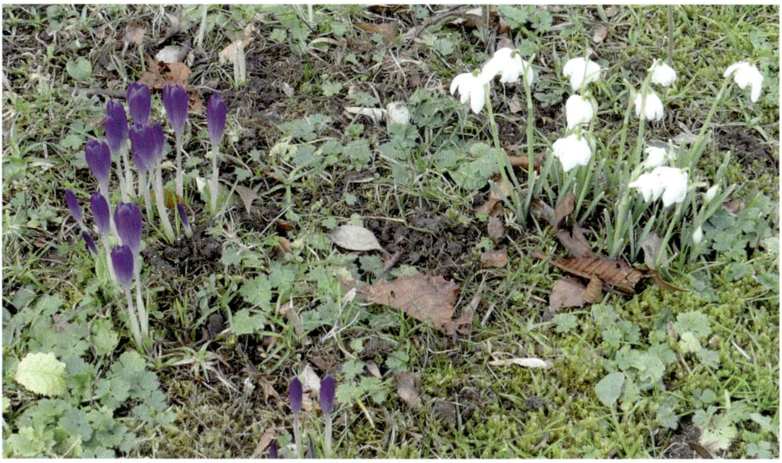

Figure 15 The common double snowdrop, *G. nivalis* 'Flore Pleno', in grass alongside *Crocus tommasinianus*, dark form.

plant to snowdrops planted in grass, as long as there is sufficient light for the Tommasini's crocus (Figure15). Dwarf varieties of the Lenten hellebore (*H. orientalis*) also flower in early spring, making them good companion plants.

A MEDICINE FROM SNOWDROPS

Galantamine, which is naturally occurring in snowdrops and daffodils, is licensed for the early treatment of symptoms of vascular and Alzheimer's dementia due to its anticholinesterase activity. This activity potentiates the action of acetylcholine, which is a key neurotransmitter required for conduction of electrical signals across synapses (junctions between nerves) in some parts of the brain and in the peripheral nervous system. Normally acetylcholine is quickly broken down by cholinesterases after its release at synapses.

Galantamine is thus a cholinergic enhancer – the idea being that the drug increases the efficacy of acetylcholine in critical parts of the brain involved in memory and cognition, two functions impaired in this disease. Although the National Institute for Clinical Excellence (NICE), which is the body charged with advising the UK's National

Health Service on medicines, has authorized the use of galantamine, it considers such medication only provides temporary improvement in countering memory loss and deterioration of cognitive functions. One criticism of the clinical trials with galantamine, and other anticholinesterases, is that they have usually been limited to a 6-month period with no later follow up.[37] NICE points out that such drugs are of limited efficacy and do not alter or slow down the course of the disease. Unfortunately, there is as yet no clinically effective cure for dementia.

THREE

MY FAVOURITE SNOWDROPS

THE FIRST THREE SNOWDROPS

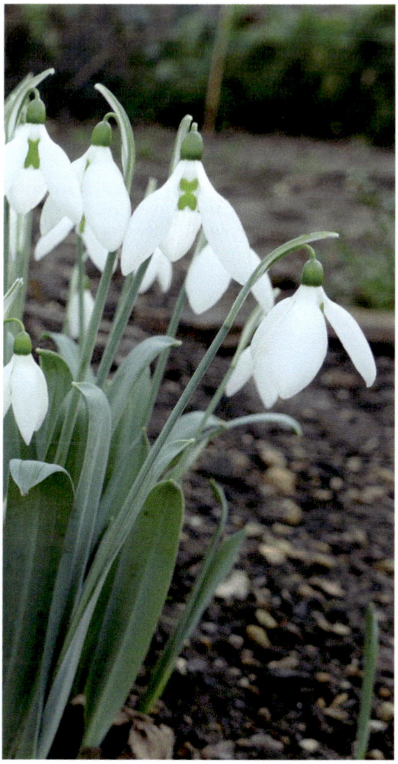

Figure 16 Group of Elwes' snowdrops (*G. elwesii*) flowering in December.

Starting a snowdrop collection can be a bit daunting. Probably the first consideration is cost. Then the question is whether you are trying to create a mass planting scheme – perhaps because you have a reasonably sized garden, or whether you just want a few choice specimens in a smaller garden.

If I had to choose three snowdrops to recommend for beginners – whether for the smaller or larger garden – I would choose the following three, which are inexpensive.

Elwes' snowdrop (*G. elwesii*, formerly *G. caucasicus*)[38] is definitely my favourite because it flowers early, between December and January (Figure 16). Elwes' snowdrop is a strong-grow-

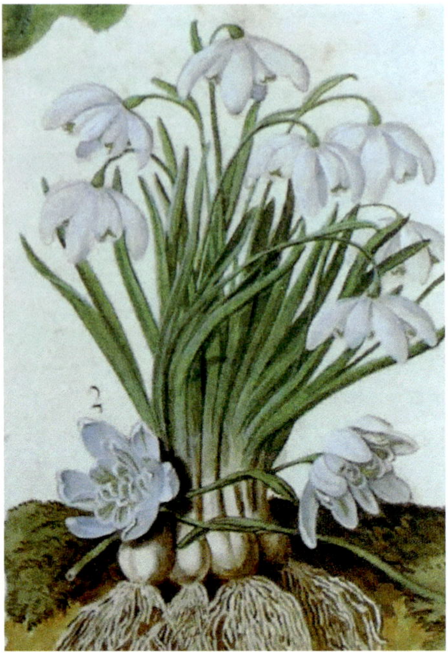

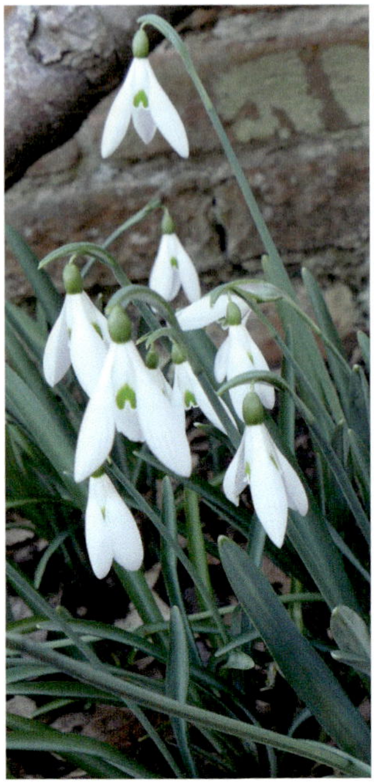

[Left] Figure 17 Common double snowdrop, *G. nivalis* 'Flore Pleno', from the Duchess of Beaufort's flowers, plate 16 (part of), Kychicus, 1703–1705 (Duke of Beaufort, 2019, with permission).

[Right] Figure 18 'Atkinsii'.

ing species and the earliest of the commonly grown snowdrops to flower. There are many fine variants usually flowering in January in the UK, although some cultivars flower at Christmas or even before. This is the best snowdrop for gardeners in my opinion, and generally has attractive glaucous-green leaves and larger flowers than the other species.

My second favourite is the standard old-fashioned double snowdrop, *G. nivalis* 'Flore Pleno'[39] because it bulks up well and is easy to grow. It will grow anywhere in the garden, including in grass, and needs little, if any, attention, except for dividing very occasionally. It flowers in January and February (Figure 17).

My third favourite is 'Atkinsii'[40] because it is tall and elegant in appearance. It usually flowers in late January and February (Figure 18).

15 SNOWDROPS FOR A GALANTHOPHILE

For a committed galanthophile, 15 snowdrops would be a good number with which to start a collection – but deciding which 15 varieties to choose is difficult because of the large number available. It is probably best visit gardens that display their snowdrop collection in February and note which varieties appeal to you.

My personal recommendations are listed in Table 2. Snowdrop varieties are listed in order of their flowering time, but these timings can differ each year according to weather conditions and their position in the garden.

My first two suggestions are the autumn-flowering Queen Olga's snowdrop (*G. reginae-olgae*) (Figure 19) and the slightly later *G. elwesii* 'Hiemalis' clone (Figure 20) that looks exactly like Elwes' snowdrop, except it emerges two months earlier in November. These are both welcome early snowdrops but are scarcely 'harbingers of spring' as winter is still to come.

Table 2 15 recommended snowdrops for the galanthophile

Species or Cultivar	Features	Flowering time
G. reginae-olgae (a)	Autumn flowering	October–November
'Hiemalis' (a)	Elwes'-type	November–December
'Faringdon Double'	Semi-double	Before Christmas
'Mrs McNamara' (a)	Tall, Elwes'-type	December–January
'Anglesey Abbey'	Green leaves	January
'Lady Beatrix Stanley' (a)	Early double	January
'Rodmarton Regulus'	Tall, large flowers	January–February
'Magnet' (a)	Nodding	January–February
'Hippolyta'	Good double	January–February
'White Swan'	Good double, elegant	January–February
'S. Arnott' (a)	Scented	January–February
'Spindlestone Surprise' (a)	Yellow	January–February
'Diggory' (a)	Attractive flowers	January–February
'Augustus' (a)	Wide leaves	January–February
G. woronowii (a)	Wide leaves	March

(a) indicates an Award of Garden Merit by the British Royal Horticultural Society.

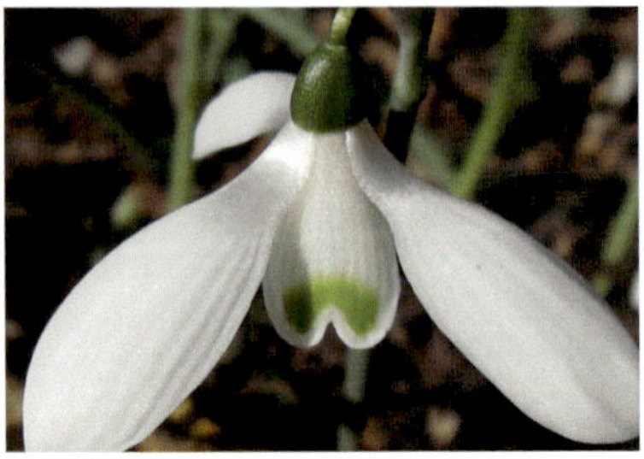

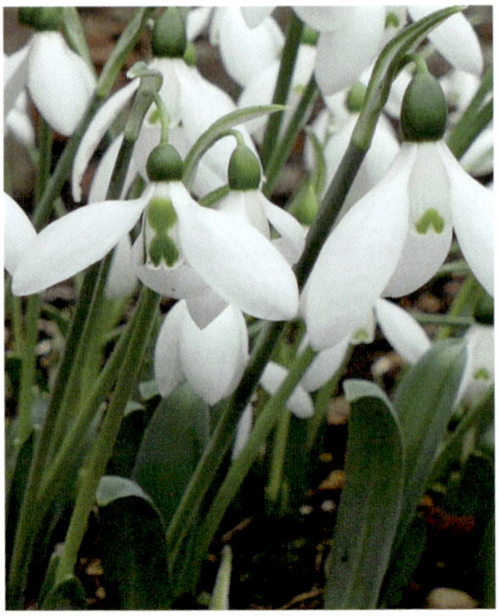

Figure 19 Queen Olga's snowdrop, *G. reginae-olgae* 'Cambridge'.

[Right] Figure 20 'Hiemalis', with different inner green markings on the two foreground snowdrops.

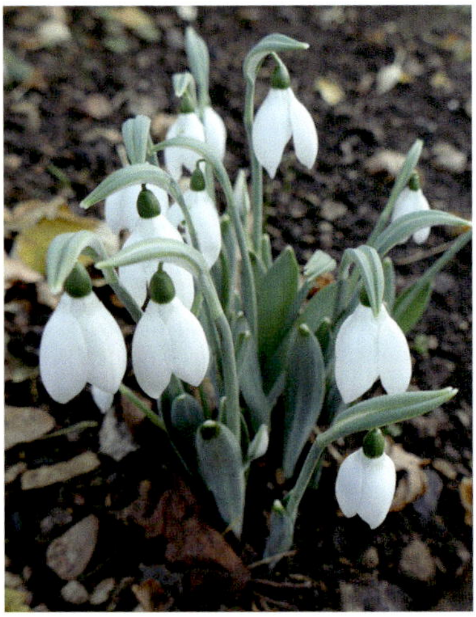

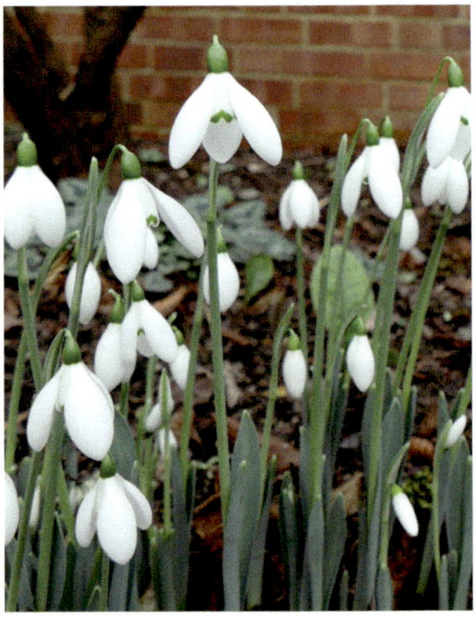

[Left] Figure 21 'Faringdon Double'. The semi-doubling is not visible in this image.

[Right] Figure 22 'Mrs McNamara'.

Two other early snowdrops are on my list and often emerge before or around Christmas. 'Faringdon Double' flowers in December and is one of the first double snowdrops to flower, although it is more correctly called a 'semi-double' (Figure 21). 'Mrs McNamara' is an extremely good, tall *G. elwesii* cultivar with large, impressive flowers. (Figure 22).

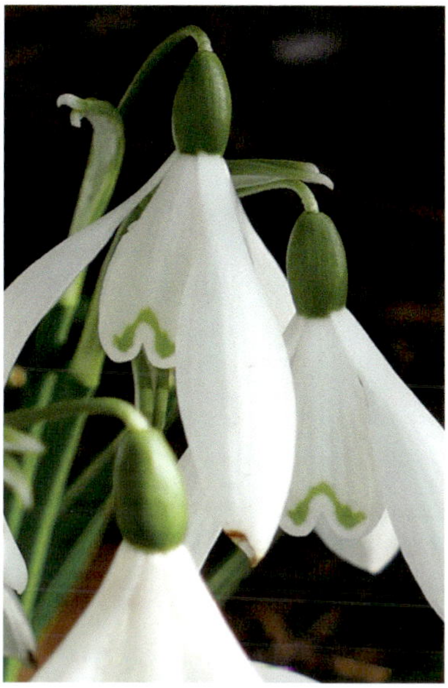

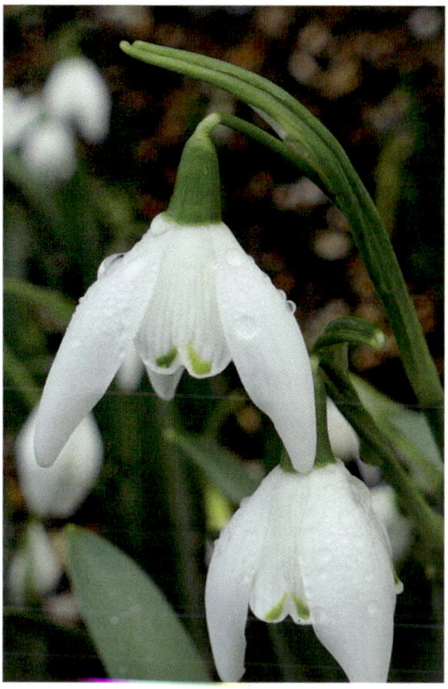

[Left] Figure 23 'Anglesey Abbey'.

[Right] Figure 24 'Lady Beatrix Stanley'.

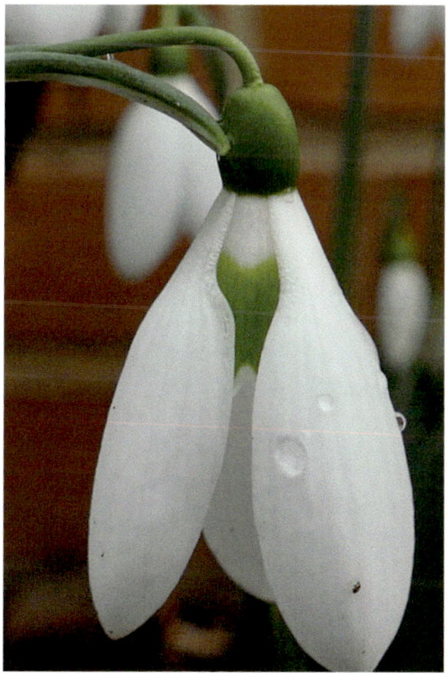

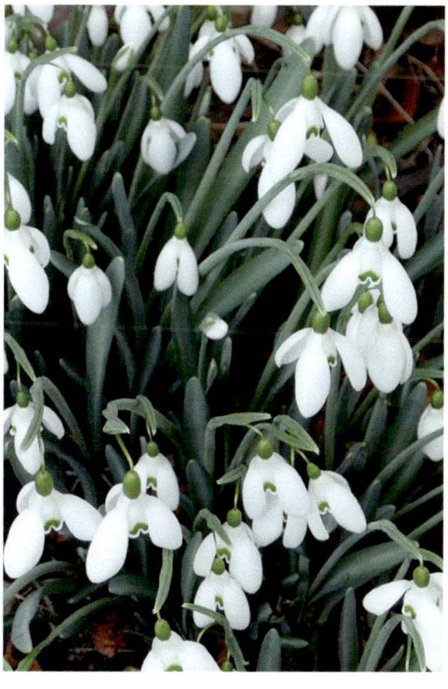

[Left] Figure 25 'Rodmarton Regulus'.

[Right] Figure 26 'Magnet'.

My next two recommendations are 'Anglesey Abbey' (Figure 23) and 'Lady Beatrix Stanley' (Figure 24). 'Anglesey Abbey', although not a large snowdrop, has distinctive, very green foliage contrasting with the more glaucous green of many of the G. *elwesii* cultivars. 'Lady Beatrix Stanley' is a very old and reliable double snowdrop. Both these snowdrops are usually out by mid-January.

Next on my list is 'Rodmarton Regulus' (Figure 25) which is the tallest growing cultivar I know of, with exceedingly large flowers, and very long, impressive leaves after flowering. I also recommend 'Magnet' (Figure 26), an old variety noted for its flowers that nod in the wind. Both these varieties are usually flowering by late January.

The hybrid 'Hippolyta' (Figure 27) is a very reliable, strong-growing double, although it does need splitting every 5–10 years. Flowering in January–February, 'White Swan' (Figure 28) is another double, which is particularly attractive because of the delayed growth of its leaves, giving it a swanlike elegance.

'S. Arnott' (Figure 29) is a classic snowdrop which has the added advantage of a good scent. Most snowdrops are scented to attract insect pollinators, but the scent is more marked in 'S. Arnott' than in most other snowdrops.

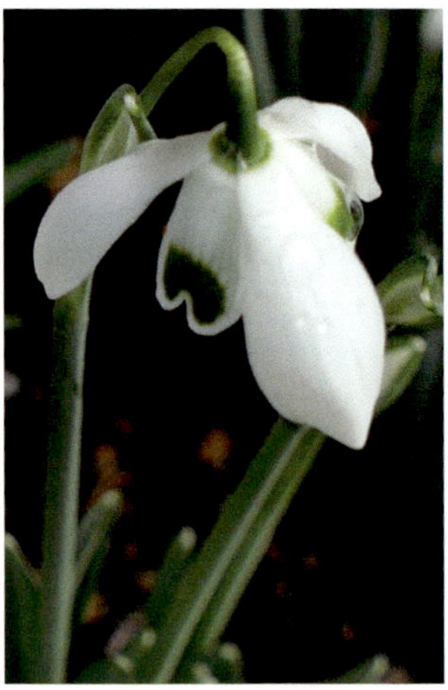

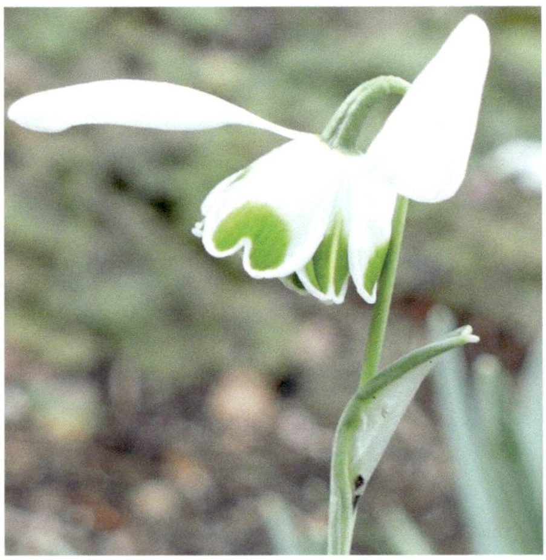

[Left] Figure 27 'Hippolyta'.

[Right] Figure 28 'White Swan'.

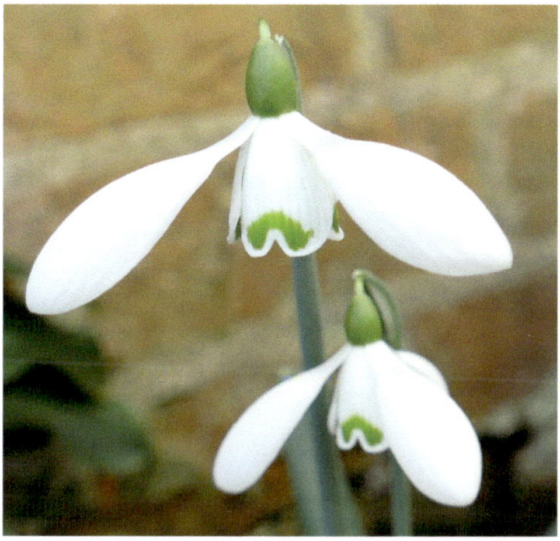

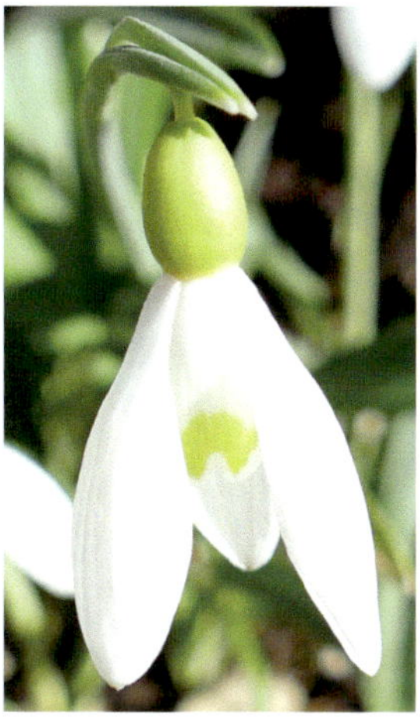

[Left] Figure 29 'S. Arnott'.

[Right] Figure 30 'Spindlestone Surprise'.

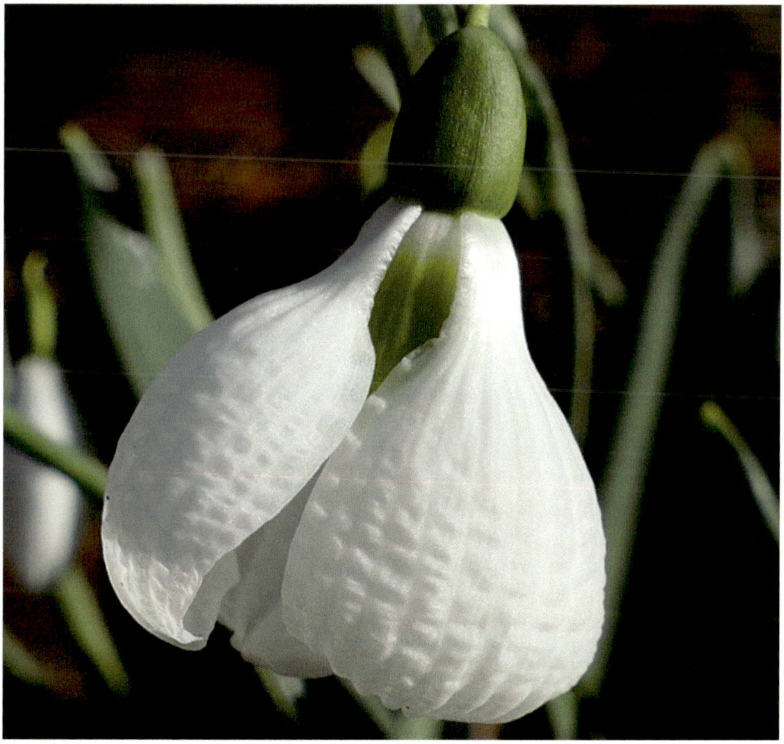

Figure 31 'Diggory'.

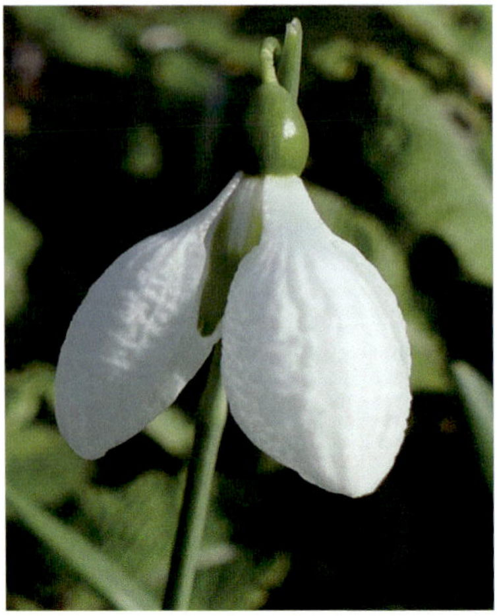

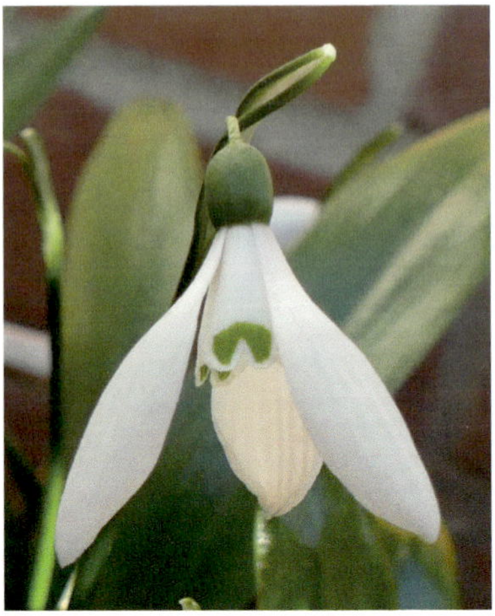

[Left] Figure 32 'Augustus'.

[Right] Figure 33 Woronow's snowdrop (*G. woronowii*), one outer petal faded.

Two rather special and more expensive snowdrops, the yellow 'Spindlestone Surprise' (Figure 30) and 'Diggory' (Figure 31), are highly recommended and flower in late January–February. 'Spindlestone Surprise' is arguable the best of the yellows and 'Diggory' is a must-have in any collection because of its very distinctive crinkly 'flat-bottomed' flowers.

Somewhat later flowering, I would recommend 'Augustus' (Figure 32) because of its distinctive wide foliage, if rather small flowers. It bulks up well and can be split easily to add to a collection.

Lastly, I recommend Woronow's snowdrop (*G. woronowii*) – a species snowdrop with wide green leaves that flowers well into March (Figure 33). This snowdrop has smallish, well-marked flowers, but its latish flowering makes it a good snowdrop for any collection. Moreover, it is inexpensive and widely available.

By growing the above varieties, you will enjoy snowdrops over a period of nearly 6 months from October to late March.

FOUR

THE SNOWDROP SEASON – AUTUMN AND WINTER

All books on snowdrop culture will include information on their approximate flowering time, whether early, midseason or late in the season. But the actual flowering time will depend on the position of planting. As with all plants, snowdrops will flower somewhat earlier in a sunny compared to a shaded position. Variation in climate conditions, which varies from year to year and is tending to be earlier each year, can also significantly influence the time of flowering. In this chapter, uniquely for a book on snowdrops, I note the time of flowering of the different varieties of snowdrops, relative to one another, in my garden in the season 2016–2017. Although snowdrops do flower at different times in different years, the order or sequence of flowering is always the same.

Snowdrops flower from October to late March or early April in the UK, depending on the variety grown. So this chapter and the following Chapter Five, 'Snowdrops in season – spring', should be of particular interest to gardeners wanting to enjoy, and perhaps extend, their collection of snowdrops to seeing them flower for 6 months of the year. Be warned, however – if you grow all the varieties mentioned, you will definitely become a galanthophile. But these two chapters contain more than the sequence of appearance of snowdrops. Snowdrops have been collected and particular cultivars named over the years because they had unusually marked flowers, or sometimes leaves or other features, e.g. yellow ovaries, distinguishing them from other known snowdrop varieties. This was often because of quirky or abnormal features such as the early named 'Scharlockii' with a split spathe and green-tipped outer flower segments, named in 1868 after the pharmacist, Jules Scharlock in Germany.[41] Many other snowdrops are named because they flower early, or their flowers are particularly large, or characteristically marked with distinguishing green markings on the inner or outer flower segments. Therefore, in describing some of the snowdrops varieties that I grow, interest is added by including the history of the name of the snowdrop, the date of naming, where the particular snowdrop described was found and any special distinguishing features of the snowdrop in question. Further details of the history of the naming of most varieties mentioned here are available in the literature.[42]

Many of the snowdrops mentioned in this chapter are illustrated, but those not shown here can be viewed in companion books,[43] or websites (see Appendix 1), which are increasingly useful for snowdrop identification. Based on my personal experience of growing snowdrops, I also highlight potential problems that can occur in any extensive collection of snowdrops, for example, difficulties in snowdrop identification, 'clonal' variation, hardiness and susceptibility to disease or predators.

4 OCTOBER

While clearing up around the mulberry tree I noticed the first sign of white on the unopened flowers of a snowdrop just peeking through the earth. This snowdrop is most unusual in flowering in autumn and was described in 1876 by the Greek botanist Orphanides, who named it G. reginae-olgae in honour of Queen Olga of Greece[44] (Figure 34), grandmother of Prince Philip, Duke of Edinburgh (1921–2021). Queen Olga's snowdrop was found in the mountains of the Peloponnesus region of Greece.

To see a snowdrop emerge in October is rather special. These early-flowering Queen Olga's snowdrops can hardly be called 'harbingers of spring' but are still welcome in autumn when many herbaceous plants have finishing flowering – even though there are many other well-known autumn-flowering bulbs. These include the yellow autumn crocus (*Ster-*

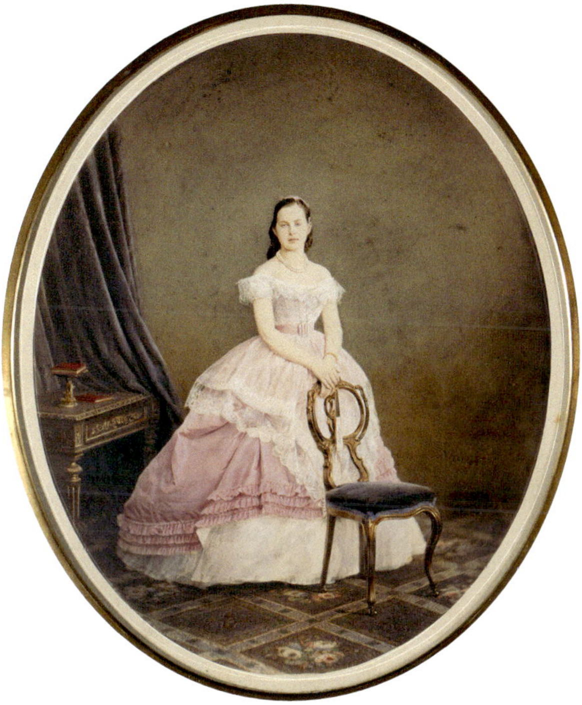

Figure 34 Grand Princess Olga Konstantinovna, Russia, 1867. Photographic portrait (with permission, The State Hermitage Museum, St Petersburg, photographer C. J. Bergamasco, salted paper print, with watercolour, © The State Hermitage Museum by Vladimir Terebenin).

nbergia lutea), and the beautiful pink or white forms of ivy-leaved cyclamen (*Cyclamen hederifolium*), as well as the true autumn crocuses and the very poisonous *Colchicum autumnale* (also known as autumn crocus) in various colours.

11 OCTOBER

The Queen Olga's snowdrops are now fully out. They look very like the familiar spring-flowering common snowdrop, *G. nivalis*, except there are no leaves visible, just the flower stem and the single white flower. Even the small, green marking on the inner flower segments looks the same as in the common snowdrop.

19 OCTOBER

We have had some more rain in the last few days and more of the Queen Olga's snowdrops have come out. Rain is needed before the autumn snowdrops emerge. When I looked today in the late afternoon, there were at least 30 flowers fully out, looking quite attractive with their ballooning outer petals.

These petals are motile – that is, they move out to open the flower and allow pollination by bees when the weather is fine, but close down to protect the flower at night in colder weather. By 7 pm, when it is dark, the petals will have closed to protect the stamens and style. Some bulbs appear to have two flower stems (scapes), which is not unusual in some snowdrops.

In two other places in my garden, more of the Queen Olga's snowdrops have now emerged but they are a week or so behind the group under the mulberry bush and are not fully out. They are also not as tall. They are different 'clones' of *G. reginae-olgae* since I obtained them from a different specialist nursery. These clones are not as robust as my other Queen Olga's clones. I maintain these different clones, but they are less vigorous than my main Queen Olga's clones for unknown reasons. As expected, none of the Queen Olga's snowdrops, despite flowering, are showing any sign of leaf yet. In these autumn-flowering snowdrops, leaves always emerge after the flowers and then grow strongly after the flowers set seed or wither.

A puzzle is why the Peshmen's snowdrop (*G. peshmenii*), which was named in 1994 after the Turkish scientist Peshmen and found on the Greek island of Kastellorizo and in southern Turkey, has failed to appear this year. It is another Mediterranean species that usually flowers a week before Queen Olga's clones. Peshmen's snowdrop is reputed to be somewhat tender, but nevertheless, it gradually formed a small clump from a single plant I purchased in 2010. It had survived several harsh winters outside with no special protection over the last 6 years and should be up by now. Perhaps, as the literature suggests,[45] it is only semi-hardy in the UK climate.

26 OCTOBER

The main group of Queen Olga's snowdrops under the mulberry bush are now looking splendid – there must be 30 or more flowers fully out. Even the Queen Olga's snowdrops in the slightly shadier parts of my garden are out, looking like vertical posts with a delicate hanging flower. The Queen Olga's snowdrops transplanted last year look surprisingly good with about 10 flowers out. This is a strong-growing, very early clone. Not all *Galanthus* clones transplant so well and flower the first year after transplanting.

30 OCTOBER

The slightly later Queen Olga's 'Cambridge' clone is now partly out (Figure 19). 'Cambridge' is a Queen Olga's clone from the University of Cambridge Botanic Garden named around 1960. It always emerges a week or two after my first Queen Olga's snowdrops and is an excellent cultivar with noticeably pointed outer petals. The spathe – a bract-like structure near the flower – is very obvious in the Cambridge clone giving the appearance of a hood over the upturned flower. The pedicel is also quite short. This contrasts with the less vigorous varieties where the spathe is not at all obvious early on. Another difference between this later flowering 'Cambridge', Queen Olga's clone and the earlier flowering clones is that about 1 cm of leaf is visible, just emerging from the ground. In addition, the ovary is bigger. All in all, the 'Cambridge' clone is a vigorous, desirable clone.

Today was warm, sunny and still, with an unseasonably high 20°C in the afternoon, and the occasional bumblebee attracted to the scent from my clump of 30 or so snowdrops. Although not that strong a scent, when I bent down to the snowdrops, I could clearly smell the same pleasant scent that was attracting the bumblebees.

Unfortunately these early snowdrops are also attractive to slugs and snails. They climb up the snowdrop at night and eat, or cut off the flower, which can be seen lying on the ground and partly eaten the next morning. They have a sweet tooth, so I placed some slug deterrent nearby. I also cleared nearby dying vegetation of herbaceous plants.

5 NOVEMBER

Clear and still dry, I decided to cut down and clear dying, herbaceous vegetation near where Queen Olga's *G. reginae-olgae* ssp. *vernalis* group (*vernalis* is Latin for spring) of snowdrops were just peeking through the earth. Subspecies *vernalis* is a recognized stable variant in the wild, hence a subspecies, differing from the Queen Olga's ssp. *reginae-olgae,* mentioned so far.[46] The *vernalis* subspecies of *G. reginae-olgae* is distinguished from the earlier subspecies *reginae-olgae* in having longer leaves at flowering time, and it also flowers later (Figure 35).

I also cut down herbaceous plants and tidied up where my 'Hiemalis' will soon flower. There are many different, very early-flowering Elwes' snowdrops (*G. elwesii*), mostly unnamed, but all are given the general name 'Hiemalis', from the Latin *hiemalis* meaning winter.

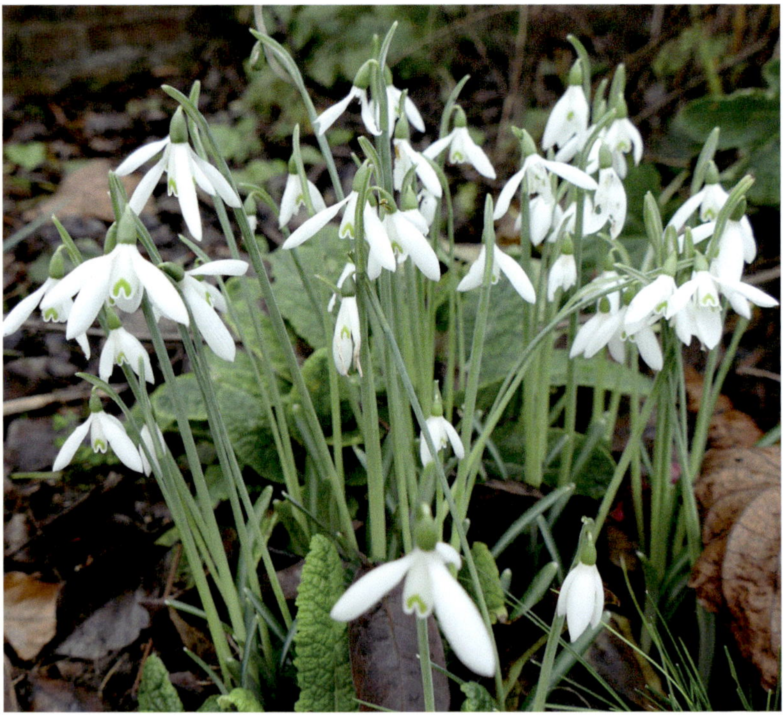

Figure 35 Queen Olga's snowdrop, *G. reginae-olgae* 'vernalis'. Note the very short leaves.

Clearing the nearby vegetation allows more sun to get to the snowdrops. I can admire them better and show them off to visitors. There is no actual sign of 'Hiemalis' yet, although the ground is still quite dry for this time of year. I bought my 'Hiemalis' from a general garden nursery as *G. elwesii*. I doubt the nursery realized they were selling me an unusual, early-flowering 'Hiemalis' snowdrop as otherwise they would have charged me much more.

17 November

We have had some rain now and one mild frost. The main group of Queen Olga's snowdrops have now been in flower for about a month. They still look nice, although a few flowers have faded. The petals have extended by growth. I had to remove several large fallen mulberry leaves which were almost covering them.

A clump of the later Queen Olga's ssp. *vernalis* snowdrops now have two flowers fully out – with 20 or so more flowers coming.

'Hiemalis' are now peeping through the earth after the recent rain. They are much later than last year when they flowered at least 2 weeks earlier.

2 December

After a lot of recent rain and two night's hard frost, the Queen Olga's snowdrops have now gone over, apart from the later flowering *G. reginae-olgae* ssp. *vernalis*. That subspecies is still not fully in flower. The other earlier Queen Olga's flowers have all set well and the seed capsules are bent over, almost touching the ground in many cases. The leaves are now very obvious, with their white central stripe – except for the weaker clones near the mulberry tree. Still no leaves are visible in that clump.

'Hiemalis' is really late this year. Two flowers in one clump are in flower, but the remaining flowers have yet to appear. Last year, in 2015, they were well out by 10 November.

10 December

We've had some milder weather – and even some sunshine – which has benefitted the snowdrops. 'Hiemalis' is now fully open (Figure 20). *G.*

elwesii was named in 1875 by Hooker after Henry John Elwes. Elwes was a plant collector and explorer who imported snowdrops from Turkey and made this species well known to gardeners. This species is generally more robust, taller and earlier to flower than the common snowdrop (*G. nivalis*). The leaves of Elwes' snowdrops are also wider, lighter green in colour and more obvious than in the common snowdrop or in Queen Olga's snowdrop.

The Queen Olga's ssp. *vernalis* group of snowdrops are now also fully in flower. Looking around my garden after clearing leaves, I noticed another white flower. This is another early-flowering cultivar, 'Faringdon Double' – a naturally occurring presumed hybrid originally discovered in the churchyard of Faringdon, Oxfordshire in 1988 (Figure 21). Naturally occurring hybrids are derived from different *Galanthus* species, but the parentage is uncertain, as in this case. It doesn't look like a double at the moment. 'Doubles' are aberrant flowers with 'doubling up' of the flower structure in quite an irregular way. But the 'Faringdon Double' is unusual amongst doubles in showing only a slight degree of doubling (Figure 36). It is generally called a 'semi-double' to distinguish it from the true doubles. When not fully open, the flower can easily be mistaken

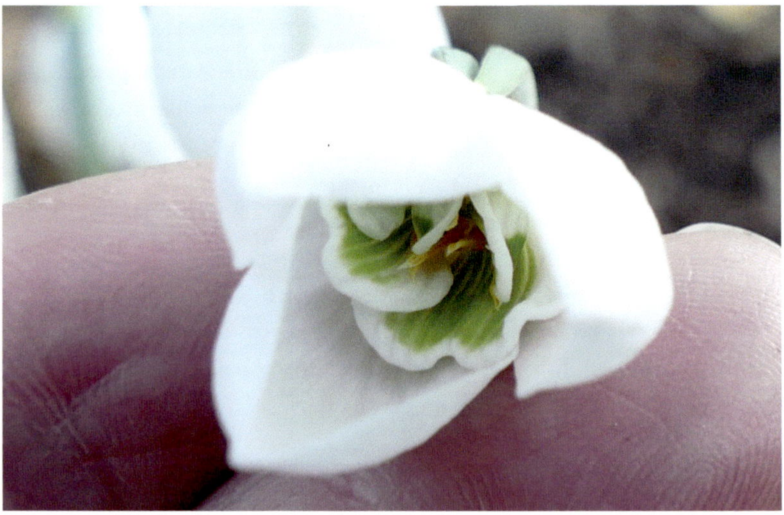

Figure 36 'Faringdon Double' flower upturned to show semi-double inside of flower.

for a normal single, but it is nevertheless very welcome as the earliest of the doubles to flower in my garden.

24 DECEMBER, CHRISTMAS EVE

The weather has continued to be unseasonably mild, giving me time over the last week to finish clearing the leaves and tidying up the borders, so I can see the green shoots of many different snowdrops beginning to emerge. 'Faringdon Double', 'Hiemalis' and Queen Olga's ssp. *vernalis* group are looking really great now.

Elsewhere in the garden, the 'Mrs McNamara' snowdrops are already quite obvious, although not yet in flower. 'Mrs McNamara' is an outstanding early snowdrop, named in 1996 by Christopher Brickell after Dylan Thomas' mother-in-law.[47] It is strong, tall and vigorous snowdrop growing up to nearly 30 cm with large, attractive flowers. Although not cheap to buy, this snowdrop multiplies well. But I had to remove some of the rather vigorous, large blue hepatica, *Hepatica transsilvanica* growing too near her.

27 DECEMBER

Today I noticed that 'Mrs McNamara' is very nearly full out in flower (Figure 22), and quite a few other snowdrops are showing a bit of white. Queen Olga's early snowdrops have mostly set seed and the leaves are now growing, except for the later subspecies *vernalis* group. The flowers of *vernalis* are just beginning to fade.

28 DECEMBER

After a heavy frost down to about –5°C last night, 'Hiemalis' and the 'Faringdon Double', which were fully out the day before, just keeled over with their flower stems (scapes) now completely bent over and covered with ice crystals and their flowers touching the frozen soil (Figure 11). They remained completely frozen and rigid all day, but always recover. How is this achieved? Snowdrops are reported to be hardy to –20°C.

Snowdrops are clearly adapted to the cold and likely have several mechanisms to protect their cells against freezing, including sugars and other chemicals that depress the freezing point of water inside cells. I have found no reference as to how snowdrops are protected from damage due to freezing, but studies in commercial crops, such as carrots and winter rye, suggest that another way plants protect themselves is by antifreeze proteins.[48] These proteins, several of which have been characterized at the molecular level, bind to ice crystals and are thought to protect against damage that would otherwise result from ice crystals. It would be interesting to determine the DNA sequence of snowdrops to discover if similar antifreeze proteins are present to those already known in other plants, or whether different antifreeze mechanisms operate.

6 JANUARY

The clump of 'Mrs McNamara' is now fully in flower, as is another early-flowering double, 'Richard Ayres', named after the head gardener at Anglesey Abbey in Cambridgeshire in 1987. It is an obvious double which has many convoluted, inner petal-like structures, some of which are irregular, but differing from the even earlier 'Faringdon' semi-double. The 'Richard Ayres' snowdrop is distinctive in having four, and sometimes more, rather obvious projecting, outer flower segments.

Also emerging is 'Wasp', discovered in 1995 by Veronica Cross.[49] It is a delicate-looking hybrid snowdrop that clumps up well, with slender leaves and a very pointed flower that resembles a wasp in flight (Figures 37, 38). It has two green marks on the inner petals, some say like a wasp's thorax, although this is a bit fanciful. Nevertheless, this is an excellent, early snowdrop.

21 JANUARY

Many snowdrops are now starting to come out but have yet still to show their full fine features. 'Mrs McNamara' is the exception. She looks splendid and some flowers within my clump stand nearly 30 cm high with their elegant, arched stems and large pendant flowers (Figure 22).

Another early double, 'Lady Beatrix Stanley', named in 1981 by Richard Nutt[50] but known since the 1950s, is now emerging (Figure

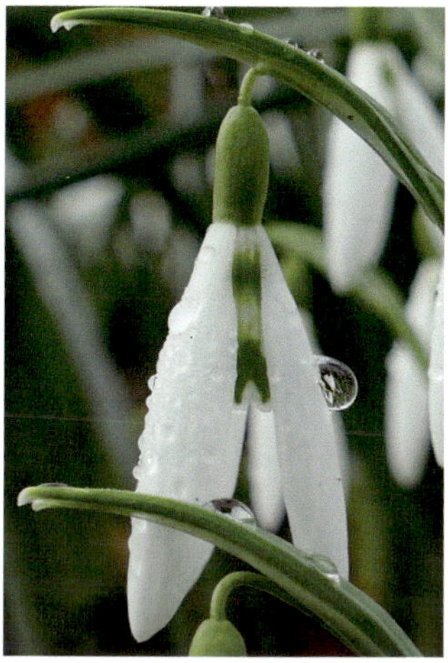

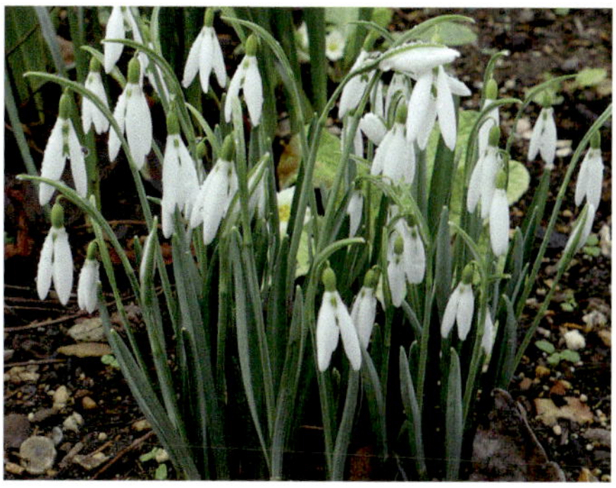

[Left] Figure 37 'Wasp'.

[Above] Figure 38 'Wasp' overview.

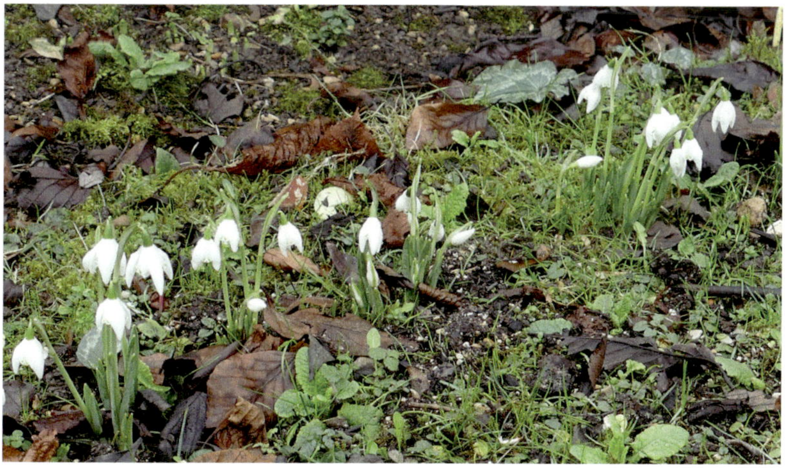

Figure 39 'Lady Beatrix Stanley' growing in rough grass near edge of lawn.

24). I have planted it in quite a few places in my garden, including in my front lawn. It seems to do well wherever it is planted. It is a rather squat snowdrop as it emerges, but then the flower stem appears to unfold and shows off its double flower, usually with irregular features and three very obvious pointed outer petals. It is a trouble-free snowdrop and has formed large clumps without the need for splitting. In the lawn, it multiplies more slowly than in the flower beds, but still comes up every year (Figure 39). It is a very reliable snowdrop.

Other doubles are not far behind. I actually started my snowdrop collection by buying the *G. nivalis* 'Flore Pleno', a double snowdrop, which explains my fascination for doubles. Doubles have been known since the early 1700s. Three of the so-called 'Greatorex' hybrid doubles are also starting to flower, although not all flowers in the clump are yet out. These are 'Hippolyta' (Figure 27), 'White Swan' (Figure 28), 'Dionysus' and 'Ophelia'. Unlike the naturally occurring hybrids mentioned so far, the 'Greatorex' hybrids were the result of deliberate crossing, over 60–70 years ago, by Heyrick Greatorex between the quite short double *G. nivalis* 'Flore Pleno' and the taller, more vigorous, wide-leaved *G. plicatus*. Heyrick Greatorex was an unconventional galanthophile but made his mark amongst snowdrop enthusiasts because he selected around a dozen such hybrids. He named them after mythological creatures or Shakespearean characters, such as 'Desdemona', 'Dionysus', 'Ophelia', 'Cordelia' (Figure 40), 'Lavinia', 'Nerissa', 'Jaquenetta', 'Hippolyta' and 'Titania' amongst others. A slightly later cross was named 'White Swan'.

These Greatorex hybrids are extremely difficult to tell apart – except for Jaquenetta, which has a much greener flower than the others. Its outer petals are usually green-tipped, which helps identification. They are extremely valuable, vigorous hybrids many of which, but not all, show almost perfect doubling and far less irregularity than the parent 'Flore Pleno' double. 'Desdemona' often produces a third leaf from a single bulb, which helps to distinguish it from the others. 'Dionysus', 'Ophelia' and 'Hippolyta' are early to flower in my garden, whereas 'Lavinia' is consistently the latest. However, this is not an absolute, as flowering can depend on the plant's position. If you plant these doubles, be sure to label the plants and keep accurate records. I keep a separate map of their positions showing exactly where I planted them. Photographs of plants in flower can also help identify their position. Be warned, birds or small mammals – and I myself when clearing leaves in the autumn – can inadvertently move plant labels.

The first of the distinctive, bright green-leaved 'Anglesey Abbey' snowdrops is also emerging (Figure 23). As its name suggests, this variant was found at Anglesey Abbey, a National Trust property near Lode, Cambridgeshire. The bright green leaves make this an easy snowdrop to identify and recognize each year. Another early-

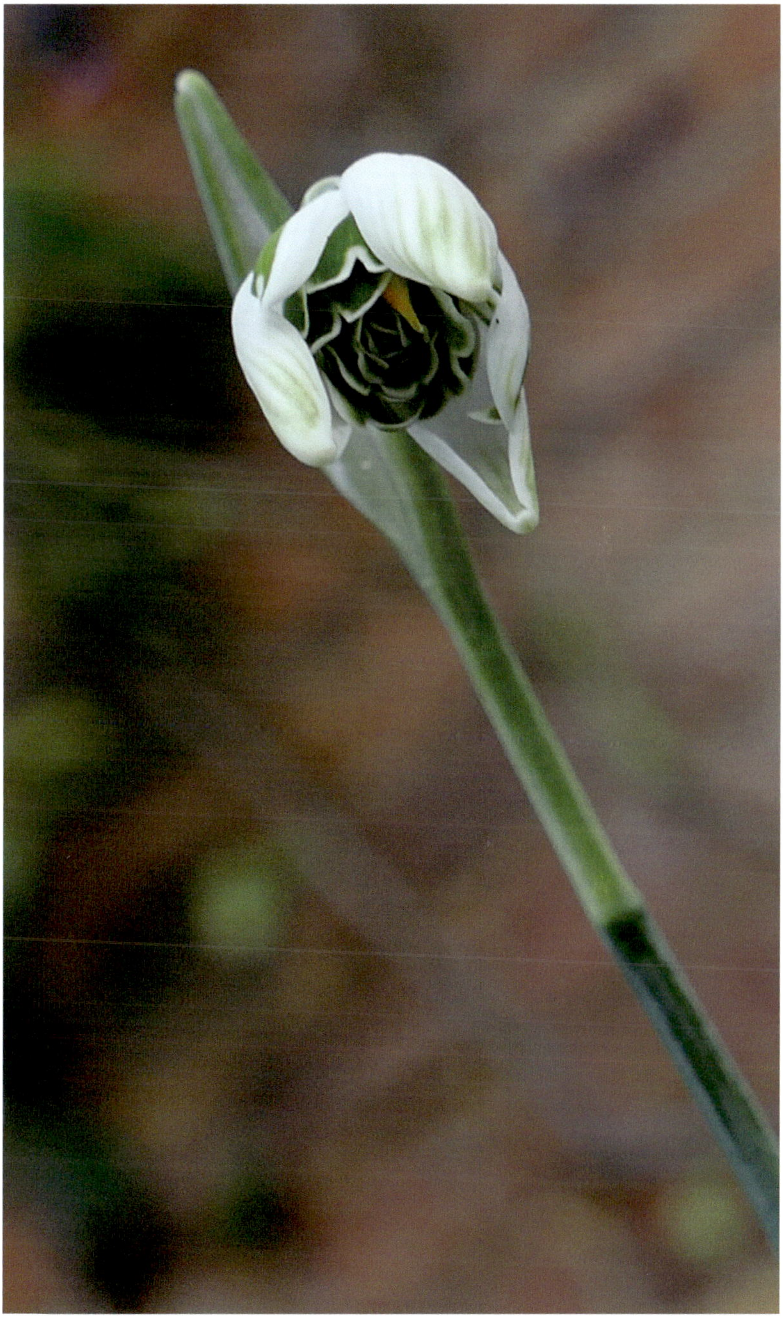

Figure 40 'Cordelia' a double snowdrop, detail.

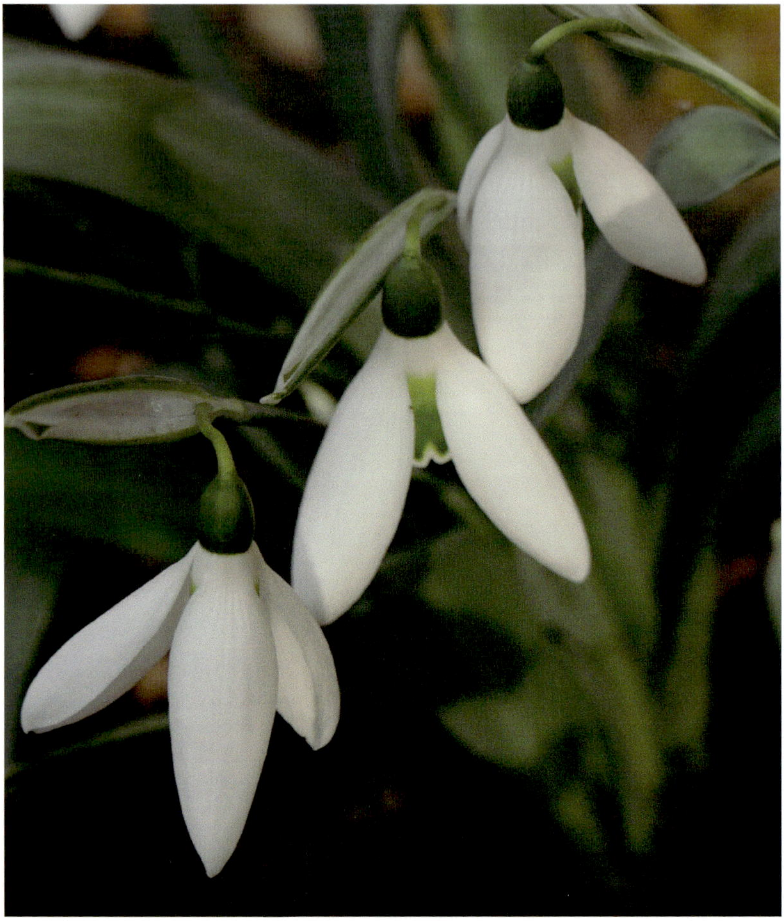

Figure 41 *G. plicatus* ssp. *plicatus.*

flowering snowdrop is 'Florence Baker'. Thought to be a *G. plicatus* clone, it has been out a week or so and has very wide leaves (3.5 cm) and impressively large flowers. The plants stand 25–30 cm tall. They have clumped up quite quickly in my garden.

Other early-flowering snowdrops – that have been out since early January – include the leafy Crimean snowdrop (*G. plicatus* ssp. *plicatus*) (Figure 41), which have smaller flowers than 'Florence Baker'. This subspecies *plicatus*, known since 1819,[51] is a classic tall, strong-growing snowdrop that does well at the back of the border.

FIVE

SNOWDROPS IN SEASON – SPRING

In this chapter I describe the order or sequence of mainly well-known snowdrop varieties coming into flower in spring 2017, following on from my description of the sequence of well-known snowdrops flowering in autumn and winter of 2016 in Chapter Four. As mentioned before, snowdrops will not flower at the same time each year because of variable weather conditions, but the sequence of flowering of different varieties will remain unaltered. The snowdrops mentioned in this chapter should be of particular interest to enthusiasts – galanthophiles – wanting to extend their collection of snowdrops. Further details of the history of the naming of most varieties mentioned here are available in the literature.[52,53,54] Many snowdrops mentioned in this chapter are illustrated, but those not shown can be viewed in companion books[55,56,57] or websites.

1 FEBRUARY

After a cold snap in January, followed by a few mild wet days, many snowdrops have just emerged. The list is long, so I will first describe my Elwes' (*G. elwesii*) snowdrops (Figure 16). They are generally tall with a glaucous (greyish green) bloom covering the leaves. They tend to flower before Christmas, but this year only a few flowers emerged early in the New Year. Most plants have been slower to flower, possibly because I divided my clump last year to swap with other enthusiasts. If one digs up snowdrops and replants, it may take a year or two for them recover and form attractive looking new clumps.

Many different cultivars of Elwes' snowdrop have been selected, particularly those with large flowers and distinctive green markings on the inner three flower segments. Even in my own garden, I have seen seedlings with different inner flower markings from my main clump. I usually keep them, marking them '*G. elwesii seedling*' and dating them the year I spotted them.

'G. Handel', named in 1986, is a Elwes'-type snowdrop that flowers quite early and has unusual light green leaves. It is said to bulk up well, but I find it is rather slow to produce offsets. Some *Galanthus* cultivars often have three leaves, as has an early Elwes'-type snowdrop, now in flower, appropriately called 'Three Leaves'. As the petals mature, they become distinctly pointed. This is another strong-growing, desirable plant. But note that a few other snowdrops, such as 'Maidwell L' and 'Robin Hood', can also occasionally boast three leaves.

Other early favourites now in flower are 'Mary Biddulph' (Figure 42), 'Maidwell L' (Figure 43) and 'Comet', which has green stripes on the outer petals (Figure 44). These three cultivars flower a bit later than my clone of *G. elwesii* and 'G. Handel'. All three are strong-growing, very large-flowered snowdrops that differ in subtle ways, such as the markings on the flowers, which can be seen if examined on one's hands and knees.

'Robin Hood' is also in flower (Figure 45). It is an older, long-established hybrid snowdrop that is very upright-looking and strong-growing and bulks up well. Some snowdrop clones split off bulbs rapidly and bulk up well, others do not. 'Little John', another vigorous, upright and tall hybrid that I acquired recently, is also now flowering.

Some of the Greatorex doubles are almost fully out and showing off their fine features. 'Hippolyta' is a very fine early double (Figure 27). 'White Swan' (Figures 28, 46), slightly later, is probably my favourite Greatorex double.

Most flowers of 'White Swan' have regular inner whorls, agreeing with Edward Augustus Bowles, who wrote in Stern's *Snowdrops and Snowflakes*:

> *'I am intensely grateful to Mr Greatorex for sending me a bulb of his new seedling, 'White Swan', which has a lovely*

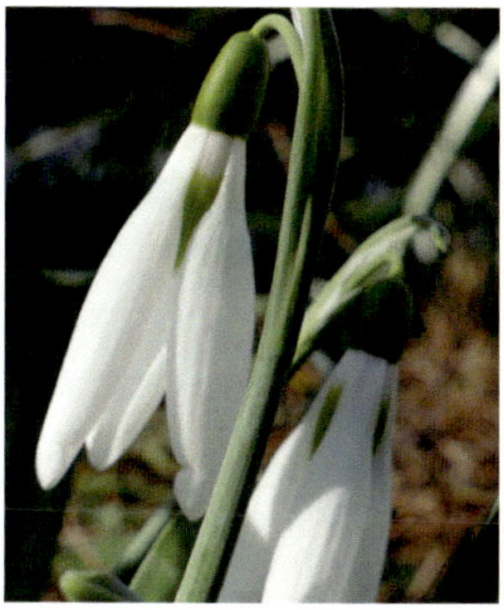

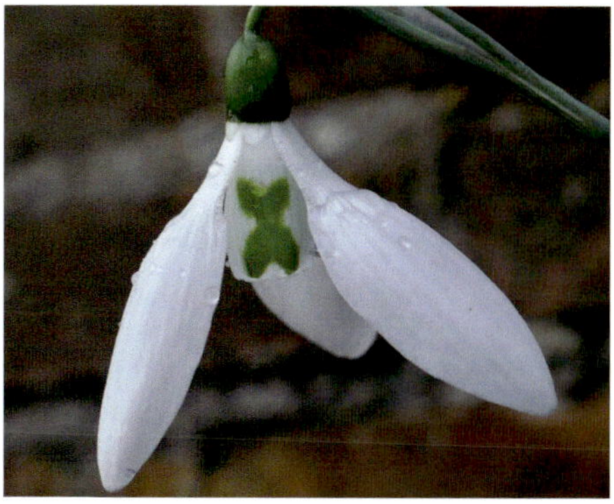

[Left] Figure 42 'Mary Biddulph'.

[Right] Figure 43 'Maidwell L'.

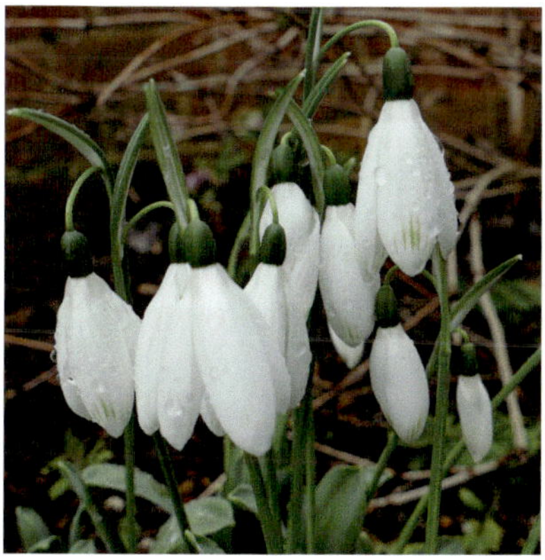

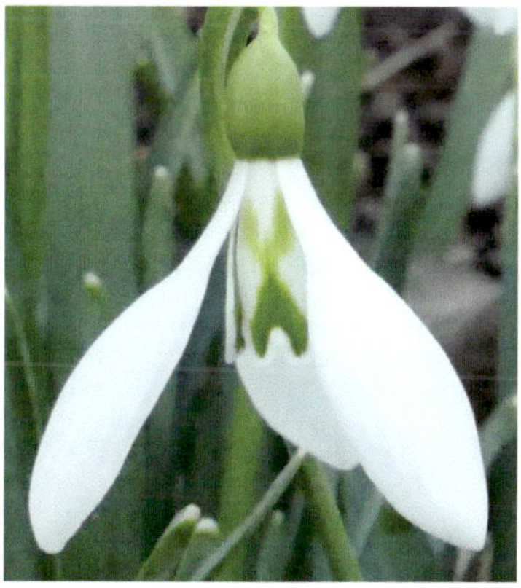

[Left] Figure 44 'Comet'.

[Right] Figure 45 'Robin Hood'.

[Below] Figure 46 'White Swan'.

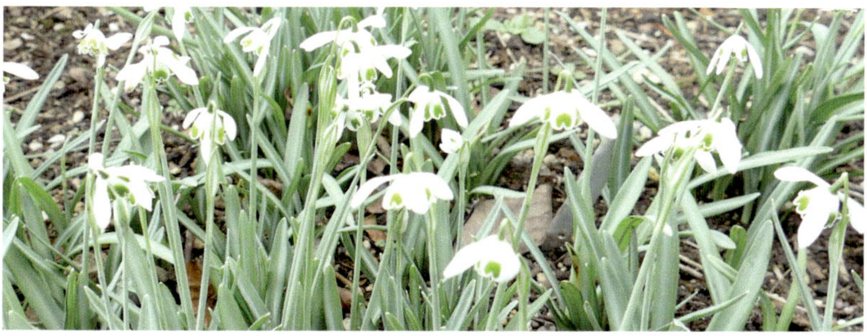

> *even rosette and massive wide outer segments, and if it will increase as happily as the others have done at Enfield it will prove one of the most precious of my snowdrop treasures and possibly the best of the doubles'.*[58]

It is possible that different, less attractive clones of 'White Swan' are in circulation because other writers[59] have not really recommended 'White Swan'.

Some of the old-fashioned, easy-to-grow and inexpensive-to-buy snowdrops are now in flower or are just coming out. 'Magnet', with its arched flowers (Figure 26), 'Atkinsii' (Figure 18) and 'S. Arnott' (Figure 29) are all well known and should be planted in every collection. 'Atkinsii' is perhaps the most vigorous of the three and occasionally produces malformed flowers. A variant of 'Atkinsii' called 'James Backhouse' also grows in my garden. All three have been available for over 50 years and are excellent single snowdrops. When the sun was shining, I saw a Painted Lady butterfly had landed on my clump of 'S. Arnott' snowdrops, presumably to collect nectar. 'S. Arnott' is reputed to be one of the most fragrant snowdrops.

A more recently described, very attractive, large and sturdy snowdrop, 'Sibbertoft Manor', is now flowering (Figure 47). It was named in 1999 by Ronald Mackenzie, who found it in the famous Sibbertoft Bank in the Oxford garden of the late snowdrop enthusiast, Primrose Warburg.

This brings me to some more doubles. 'Ballerina' is now in flower, named in 1991. She lives up to her name when the sun allows the flower to fully open like a ballerina. Another double is 'Natalie Garton' – the only double Elwes'-type *G. elwesii* snowdrop that I grow. I would describe this snowdrop as a semi-double similar to 'Faringdon Double'. It has the broad, glaucous green leaves typical of *G. elwesii*. 'Rodmarton' is another, very green double, which is only subtly different from the Greatorex 'Jaquenetta' and named because of its origin at Rodmarton Manor in the Cotswolds. It is now flowering.

Three other Rodmarton snowdrops, all singles, are definitely worth growing. 'Rodmarton Regulus' is a very impressive tall plant (25–30 cm) with huge flowers and large leaves (3 cm wide) – now fully out. It is not registered[60] but is, nevertheless, very desirable (Figure 25). The

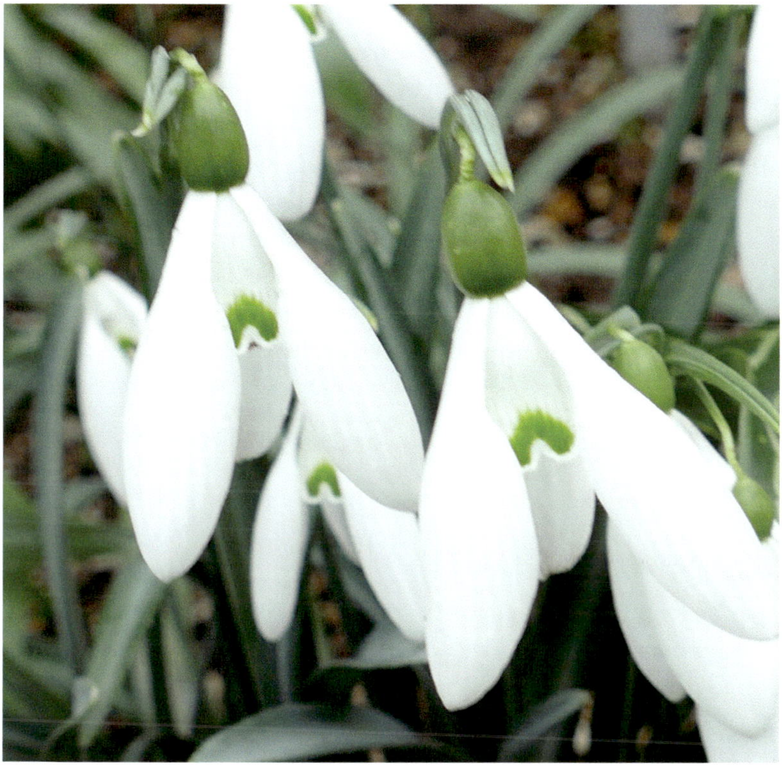

Figure 47 'Sibbertoft Manor'.

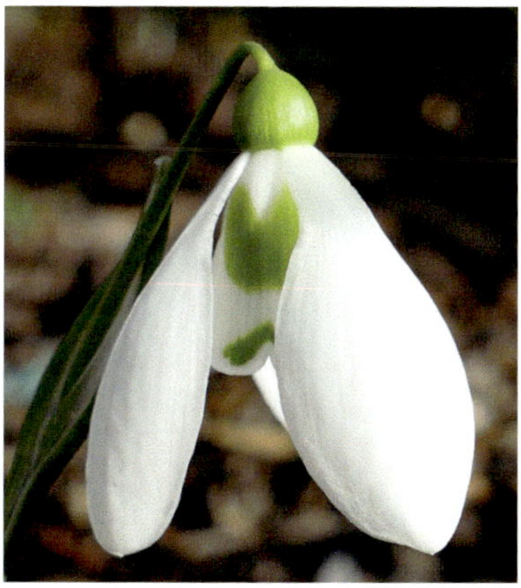

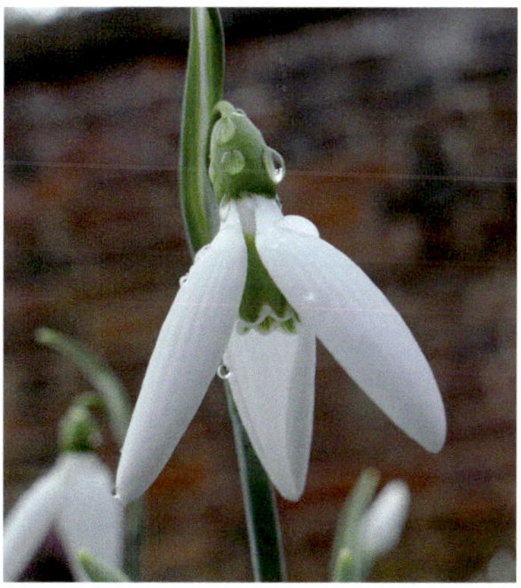

[Left] Figure 48 'Rodmarton Sirius'.

[Right] Figure 49 'Rodmarton Capella'.

other two, 'Rodmarton Sirius' (Figure 48) and 'Rodmarton Capella' (Figure 49), are shorter Rodmarton-selected variants, with large flowers and leaves, that are just coming into flower.

Some of the more unusual snowdrops are in flower now. Snowdrops, to the casual observer, are often boring because they are just tiny, white-flowered plants. Red or blue snowdrops are not known, although it is not impossible that someone will engineer these colours into snowdrops one day. But 'yellows' – with yellow ovaries and yellow markings on the flowers – are well known and are desirable snowdrops for the collector who wants to extend their range of snowdrops. The first of my yellows to flower, 'Wendy's Gold' (Figure 50) and 'Spindlestone Surprise' (Figures 30, 51) are flowering now. My clone of 'Wendy's Gold' appears to be virus-infected, producing distorted often yellow-tinged leaves but is still highly desirable.

'Diggory', another distinctive snowdrop, is flowering now. It is an immediately recognizable Crimean snowdrop, G. *plicatus*-type, because of its ballooning, crinkled flower (Figure 31). When first introduced in 1998, its bulbs commanded very high prices. Not quite so highly prized, but equally distinctive is 'Blewbury Tart' – originally found by Alan Street in the churchyard in the village of Blewbury, Oxfordshire. It is an odd-looking, very green double with upward rather than the usual downward hanging flowers (Figure 52). I place 'Diggory' and 'Blewbury Tart' at the front of a border where they can be easily seen and hopefully admired.

Two other more old-fashioned, medium-sized snowdrops are in flower. They are 'Winifrede Mathias', found in the 1950s and named after the snowdrop enthusiast Mrs Mathias, and 'Daphne's Scissors', named after Daphne Chappell, who found this snowdrop in 1985 as a green-tipped *G. elwesii* variant. My clone, surprisingly, lacks these characteristic green tips but has the scissor-shaped green markings in the inner petals. Perhaps 'Daphne's Scissors' will show green tips in future years, as green tips in snowdrops are known to be a variable feature.

The slender snowdrop *G. gracilis* 'Highdown' is another cultivar that is just coming into flower but has not been mentioned so far. It, and other *G. gracilis* variants, usually have narrow, somewhat twisted,

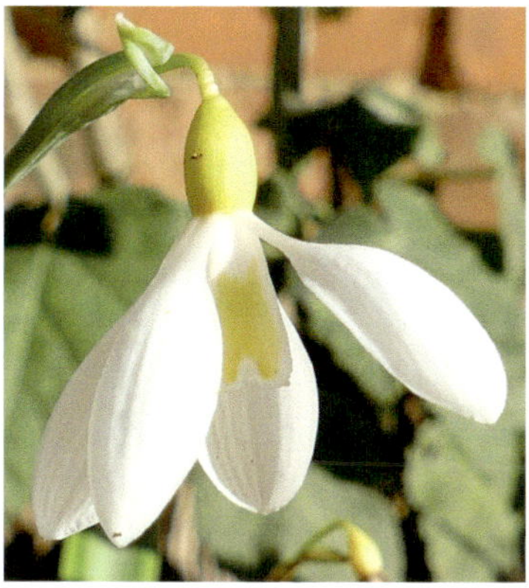

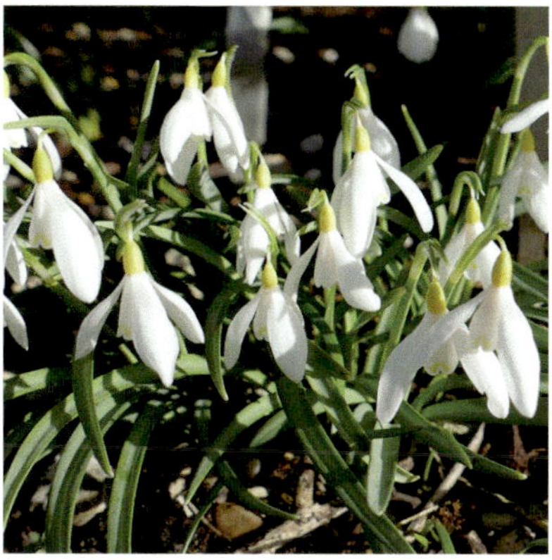

[Left] Figure 50 'Wendy's Gold', unusually with four outer petals.

[Right] Figure 51 'Spindlestone Surprise'.

[Below] Figure 52 'Blewbury Tart'.

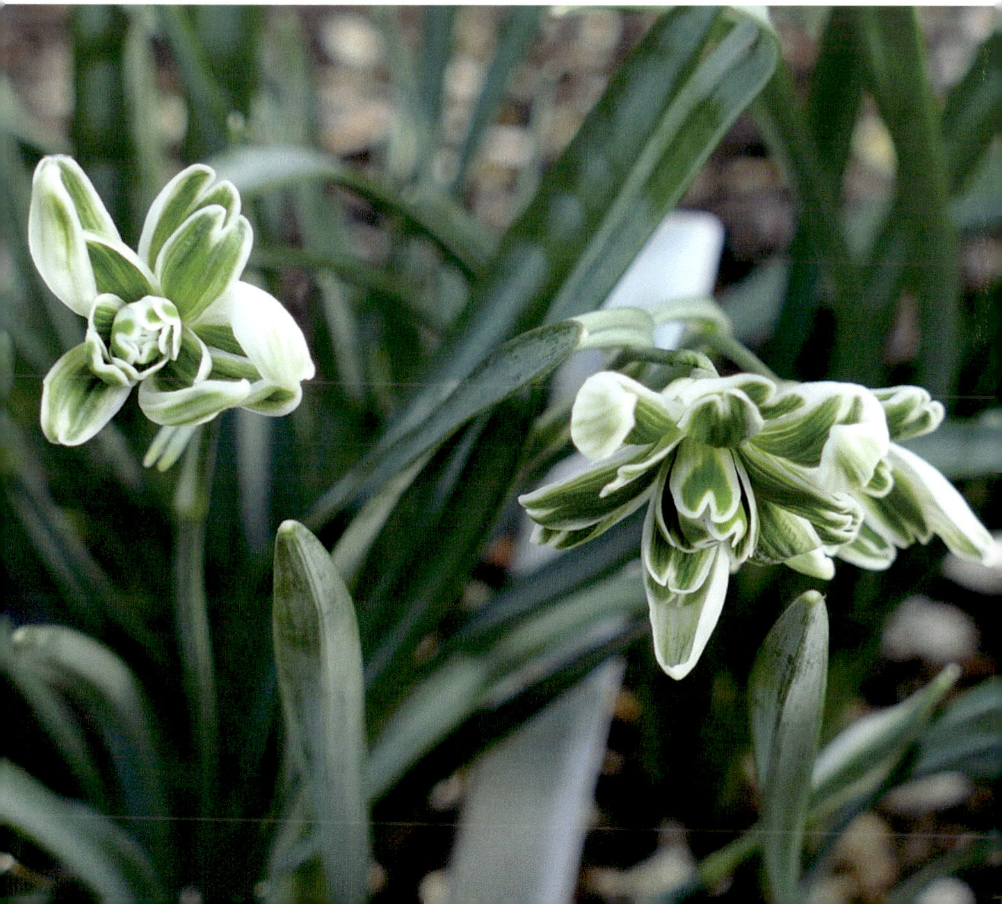

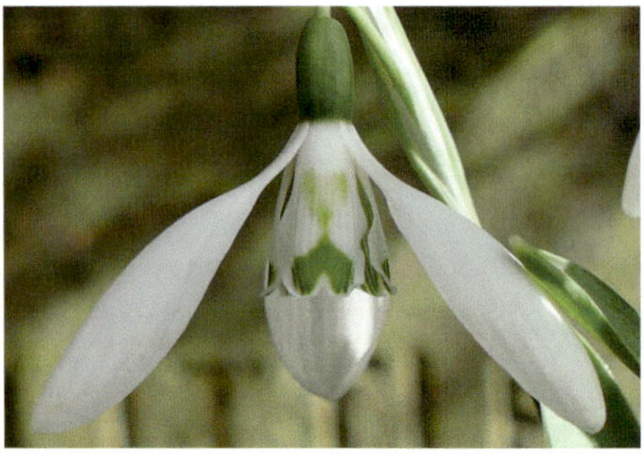

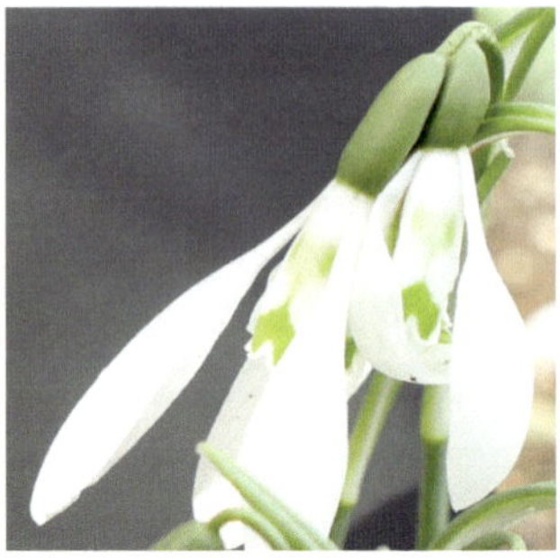

[Left] Figure 53 'Kite'.

[Right] Figure 54 'Kite', with aberrant twinned ovaries.

grass-like leaves and characteristic strong green markings on the inner flower.

Another snowdrop, 'Kite', is just emerging (Figure 53). It is a strong-growing, attractive snowdrop looking somewhat like a kite when fully open in the sun – although we have had precious few sunny days recently. I did not realize until last year that 'Kite' occasionally produces aberrant double or twinned ovaries, with two flowers each co-pressed (pressed against one another) and looking extremely odd (Figure 54). This year I cannot see any aberration on either of my clumps of 'Kite'. So, in my experience, this double ovary aberration occurs only occasionally.

Aberrations are a well-known feature of 'Mrs Thompson', another snowdrop I have grown successfully for more than 10 years, but one which I lost last year, inexplicably. 'Mrs Thompson' is perhaps the best known of all the aberrant snowdrops, producing all sorts of distinctly odd features (Figure 55), such as variable number of outer petals (up to six), ovary doubling and even normal-looking flowers. I have now bought two replacement plants at vast expense (£27 each) as this is a must-have plant. Mrs Thompson from Escrick in Yorkshire found this freakish plant around 1950, so it is now quite a well-known variant.

This brings me to the subject of why I, and other snowdrop enthusiasts, lose snowdrops from time to time. One obvious reason is that not all snowdrops are fully hardy. Frost could have been the reason for the demise of my Peshmen's snowdrop (*G. peshmenii*) as this species is said to be tender.[61]

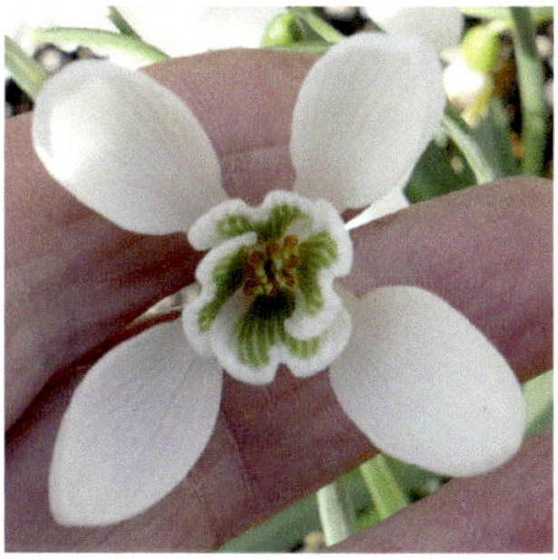
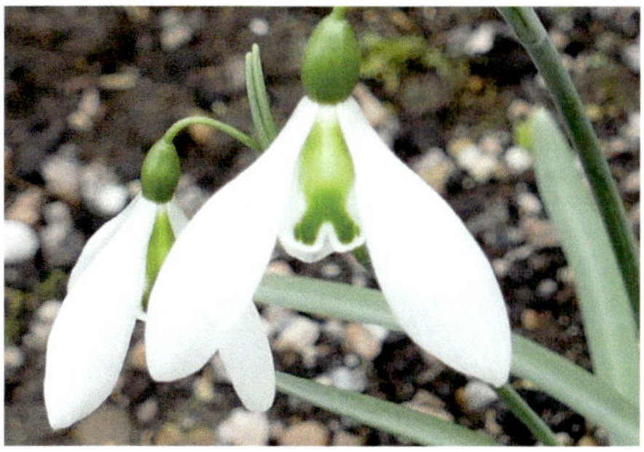

[Left] Figure 55 'Mrs Thompson', with four aberrant inner and outer petals.

[Right] Figure 56 'John Gray'.

However, this cannot be the reason I have lost other cultivars, such as 'John Gray', which is quite hardy (Figure 56). It is possible that the bulbs dried out in summer, as they were planted in a very warm, sunny situation near a dry wall. Snowdrop bulbs are known to be susceptible to drying out.[62] However, this is speculation and, equally possible, they could have succumbed to disease from fungal or insect pathogens, as discussed in Chapter Two. 'John Gray' is a vigorous tall, well-marked snowdrop named after the snowdrop enthusiast of the same name in the 1960s. This cultivar has large flowers on long flower stems so that flowers often droop down touching the earth, making them vulnerable to slug, fungal and rain damage. One fungal disease, *Botrytis*, has definitely caused losses of my slender snowdrop *G. gracilis* 'Highdown'.

9 FEBRUARY

During this last week, the milder, wetter weather has brought most of my snowdrops out, with the exception of a few late ones. Snowdrops grow with amazing speed at this time of year – but they need sun to be seen at their best and the sun is sadly lacking this week.

Let me start with some more snowdrops not yet mentioned. 'Straffan', a classic Irish snowdrop, is well out now (Figure 57). It is a Crimean snowdrop, *G. plicatus*-type, with largish, rounded flowers. It commonly, but not always, produces two flower stalks from one bulb. Indeed, this is why it was selected in the late 1800s.

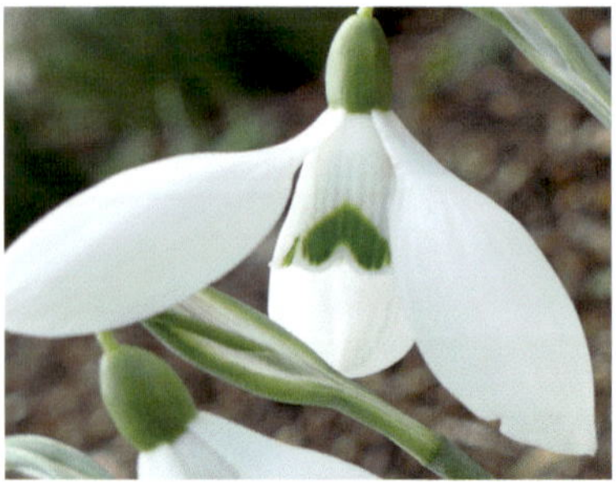

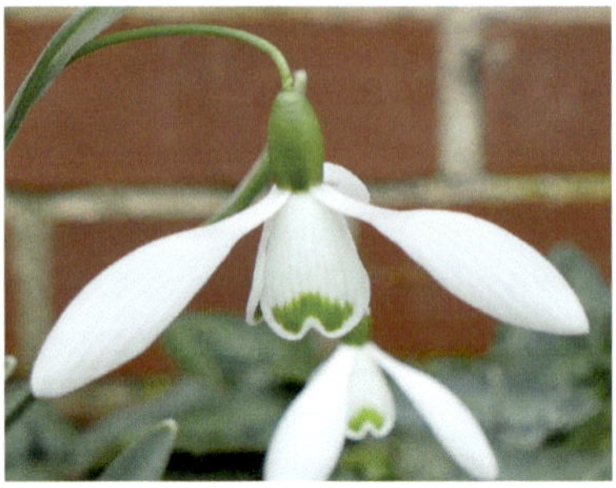

[Left] Figure 57 'Straffan'.

[Right] Figure 58 'Galatea'.

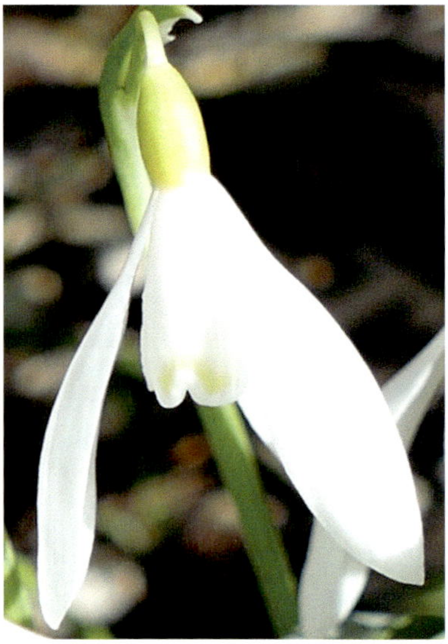

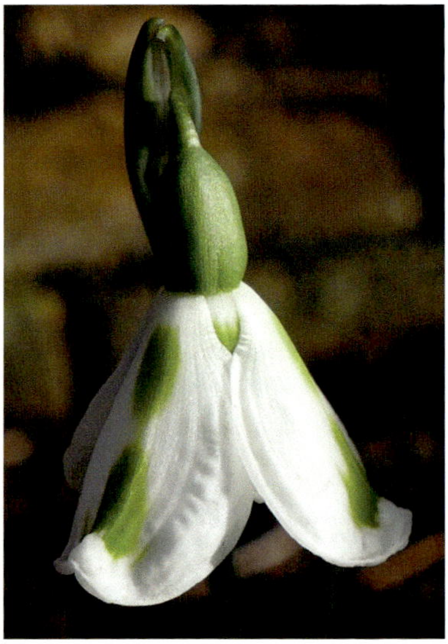

[Left] Figure 59 'Sandersii'.

[Right] Figure 60 'Trimmer'.

'Galatea' is another good snowdrop with a long flower stalk, like 'Magnet', but differs in that it is usually kinked.[63] Although named in 1891, the modern stock is believed to have arisen from stock rediscovered in the 1970s (Figure 58).

Another of my yellow snowdrops is in flower. It is 'Sandersii', named after Mr Sanders of Newnham, Cambridge, who found it in

Northumberland. It is a decidedly dwarf variety, but charming and, in 1876, was the first of the yellows to be named. According to Davis,[64] it is a delicate snowdrop and not easy to grow (Figure 59). Indeed, I have lost a clump of 'Sandersii' that I planted in other places in my garden in the past, but my present clump – underneath an *Abutilon* bush and in some shade in the summer – seems to be doing well.

Two other unusual snowdrops are now flowering, 'Trimmer' (Figure 60) and 'Godfrey Owen'. 'Trimmer' is an earlier flowering seedling of 'Trym' (not yet flowering). Both 'Trym' and 'Trimmer' are unusual, but very desirable, snowdrops with shorter outer petals (resembling a Chinese pagoda), marked with green – quite different in appearance to other snowdrops. 'Godfrey Owen', named in the mid-1990s, is the other unusual snowdrop, now flowering. It has six outer petals, as well as six inner ones, giving it a sturdy and spreading appearance.

Another quite normal-looking snowdrop, but one with very distinctive spreading leaves, 'Augustus', is now in flower (Figure 32). It was named in 1976 after the famous snowdrop enthusiast Edward Augustus Bowles. This is a dwarf Crimean *G. plicatus*-type snowdrop. The leaves are characteristically oval in appearance, quite wide and with an obvious central white stripe, making this snowdrop easily recognizable. Virus-free clones are available, although mine is probably potyvirus-infected because it occasionally shows yellowing and misshapen leaves. The flowers are not huge but display some crinkling, as seen in 'Diggory' and other snowdrops. 'Augustus' is an attractive, vigorous and useful snowdrop.

Another Crimean *G. plicatus*-type snowdrop flowering now is 'Warham', an old variety possibly introduced from Crimea in 1855. It is vigorous with broad leaves and a stripe on the upper surface – not unlike 'Augustus' – but with more upright leaves.

Other distinctive snowdrops flowering include 'Bertram Anderson' and 'Brenda Troyle'. 'Bertram Anderson' has large flowers and is quite tall. 'Brenda Troyle', by contrast, is an older snowdrop of medium size coming out a bit later than 'Bertram Anderson'. 'Benhall Beauty' is another tallish snowdrop, an older variety, named in 1961 that I grew for many years, but has also unaccountably disappeared from my garden. To my surprise, on visiting my late son's grave later in March,

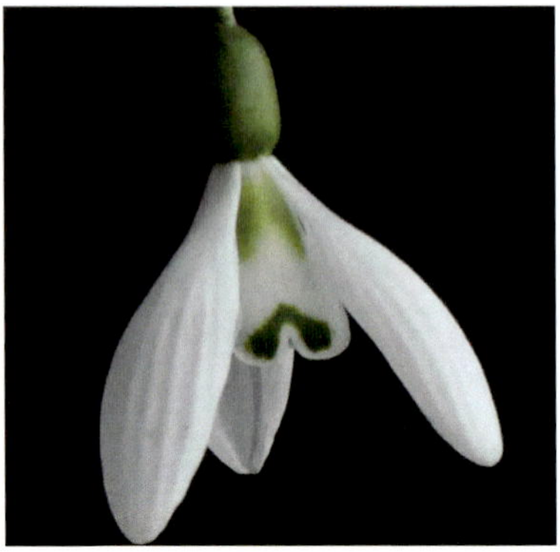

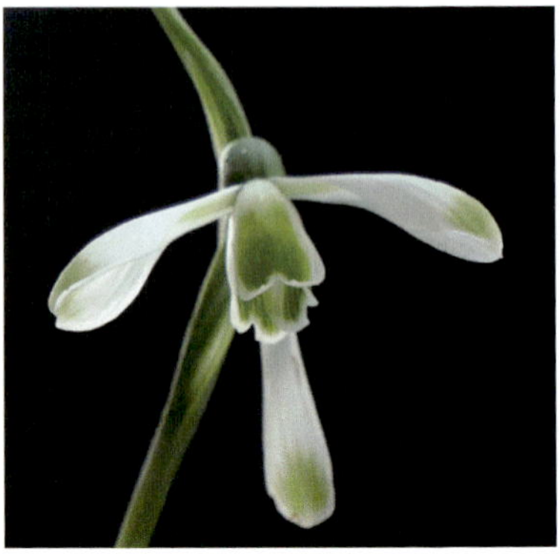

[Left] Figure 61 'Benhall Beauty'.

[Right] Figure 62 'Modern Art'.

I discovered a healthy clump of 'Benhall Beauty' in flower with its unmistakable distinctive inner segment markings and a good scent (Figure 61). I had forgotten I had transplanted some bulbs there some 10 years before.

The moral is always to divide up a new snowdrop clump as soon as possible, and plant in more than one place to guard against loss.

14 FEBRUARY (VALENTINE'S DAY)

This date reminds me that the snowdrop was deemed to be an emblem of feminine purity – one of its old names being 'Fair Maid of February'.[65] Most snowdrops are now flowering and look good in the afternoon sun. I will first mention the ones most liked by visitors. Everyone admires the large size of 'Rodmarton Regulus' (Figure 25) and the smaller but distinctive 'Wasp' (Figure 37). 'Diggory' (Figure 31) is always noticed because of its unusual flowers, and 'Augustus' (Figure 32) is liked because, though smaller in size, it has very attractive, unusual leaves. The yellow-flowered 'Spindlestone Surprise' (Figure 30) looks good now. Visitors also notice an extensive group of 'White Swan' (Figure 46) and 'Lady Beatrix Stanley' (Figure 39) that I grow in the lawn. They stand out well in my rather mossy, unfertilized and untreated lawn.

Let me now mention snowdrops newly out. 'Modern Art' is a strong, very upright, green-tipped snowdrop that was introduced, it is believed, around 1960 (Figure 62). It is distinctive and worth growing, as is 'Scharlockii', another rather strange looking snowdrop of which I have two clones. Named after a Julius Scharlock in 1868, one clone is now out. The other, a weaker clone, has still to flower. 'Scharlockii', usually green-tipped, differs from other snowdrops in that the spathe (the original membranous covering of the flower) splits into two separate long and curved green leaf-like structures, giving it an unusual appearance. Some say it resembles miniature, elongated donkey's ears.

'Washfield Colesbourne' is another very elegant snowdrop with strong green markings covering most of the inner petals. It is said to be a seedling of the much more difficult, 'Colesbourne'. When the weather is sunny, a clump of this snowdrop looks exceptionally fine. Unfortunately, my clone is only slowly producing offsets, so I have been unable to split my clump, even though I have had it for over 7 years. Maybe I should now divide 'Washfield Colesbourne' in the hope that it might grow better somewhere else in my garden. That is the general advice when snowdrops seem not to be thriving.

'Merlin' is another classic snowdrop just now coming into flower. It has been known since the 1890s and has very full green inner markings, although the flower is not large by modern standards. However, it has not been as strong growing as some other old favourites in my garden, such as the 'Greatorex' doubles or 'Galatea' that I grow nearby.

Another common snowdrop (*G. nivalis*) variant, 'Warei', has come out (Figure 63). Originally thought to be a seedling of 'Scharlockii' because of its long, elongated spathe, it is quite small with green-tipped flowers and a very long pedicel that droops in a characteristic way. My clone is small and, unusually, has split spathes, like 'Scharlockii'. It should be planted near the front of a border. Another diminutive, later double, 'Barbara's Double', is now flowering. It is said to have almost perfect doubling with no aberrant features. While I like this double, it is difficult to maintain because it is not as strong growing as the later Greatorex doubles, such as 'Nerissa', now in flower, or 'Lady Beatrix Stanley', still flowering. 'Barbara's Double' is definitely only for the specialist grower.

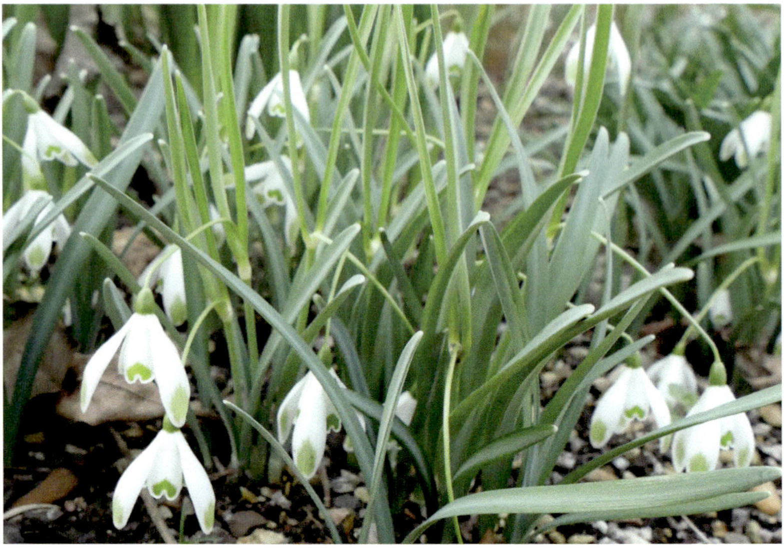

Figure 63 'Warei'.

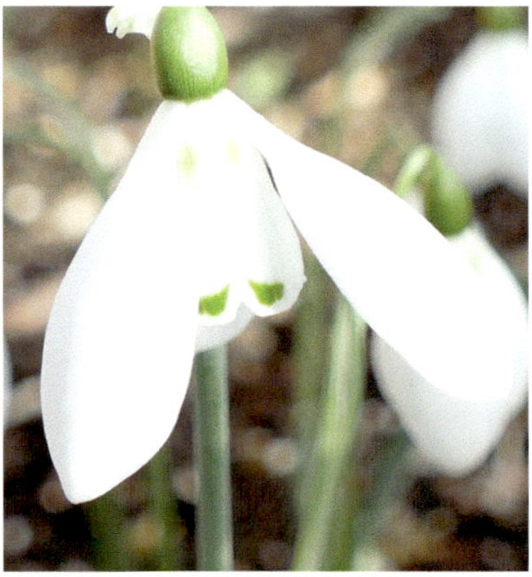

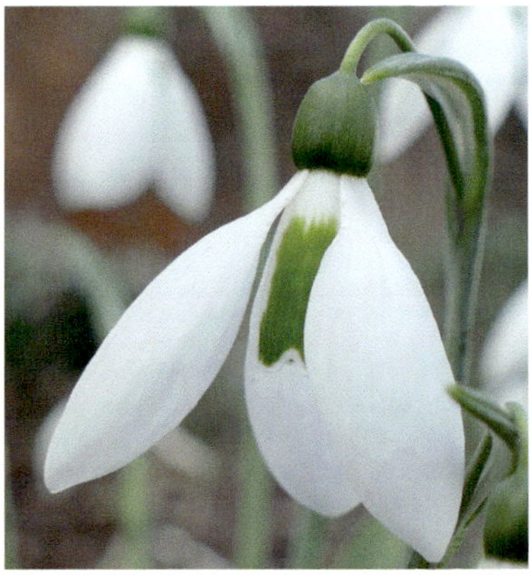

[Left] Figure 64 'Ketton'.

[Right] Figure 65 'Abington Green'.

Other snowdrops now in flower are 'Ketton' and 'Abington Green'. Both are desirable, strong-growing and distinctive varieties. 'Ketton', named in 1948 after the village of Old Ketton near Peterborough, has unusual markings on the inner parts of the flower (Figure 64).

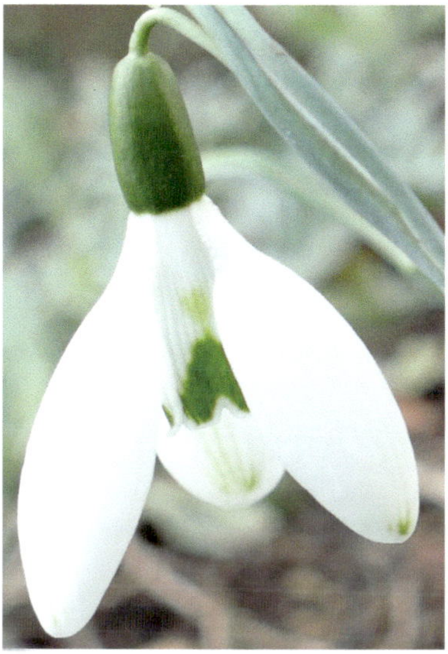

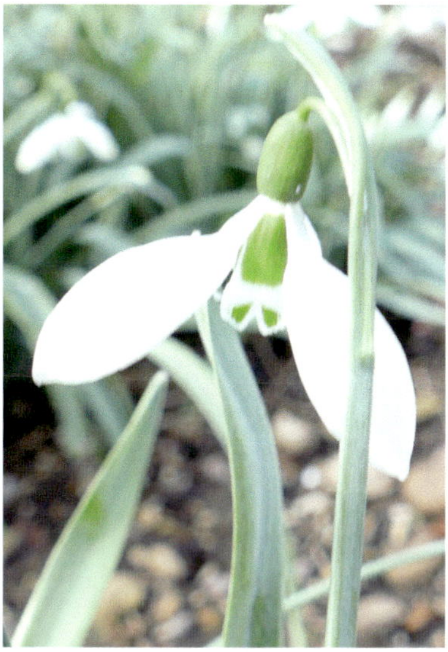

[Left] Figure 66 'Cedric's Prolific'.

[Right] Figure 67 'Daglingworth'.

'Abington Green' was discovered later in the 1970s in Little Abington, Cambridgeshire, and has bold green markings on the inner perianth segments (Figure 65). 'Cinderdine', like 'Abington Green', is an Elwes'-type G. *elwesii* snowdrop. It was found in 1996 and has largish flowers compared with the overall size of this plant – the outer perianth segments are likened to a boat. Two other quite modern Elwes'-type snowdrop variants flowering now are 'Yvonne Hay' and 'Cedric's Prolific' (Figure 66). 'Cedric's Prolific' was found in the Benton End garden of the plantsman Cedric Morris and named after him. Both cultivars have wide, glaucous green leaves and attractive, large flowers with good bold, inner markings.

'Daglingworth' is now flowering (Figure 67). It is a strong, upright snowdrop with distinctive inner flower markings, typical of the markings seen on the slender species snowdrop, *G. gracilis*. This is a very good snowdrop to have in one's garden.

'Mighty Atom' is now out forming a good clump (Figure 68). It is an old favourite with large flowers, as is 'Tubby Merlin'. Both belong to the

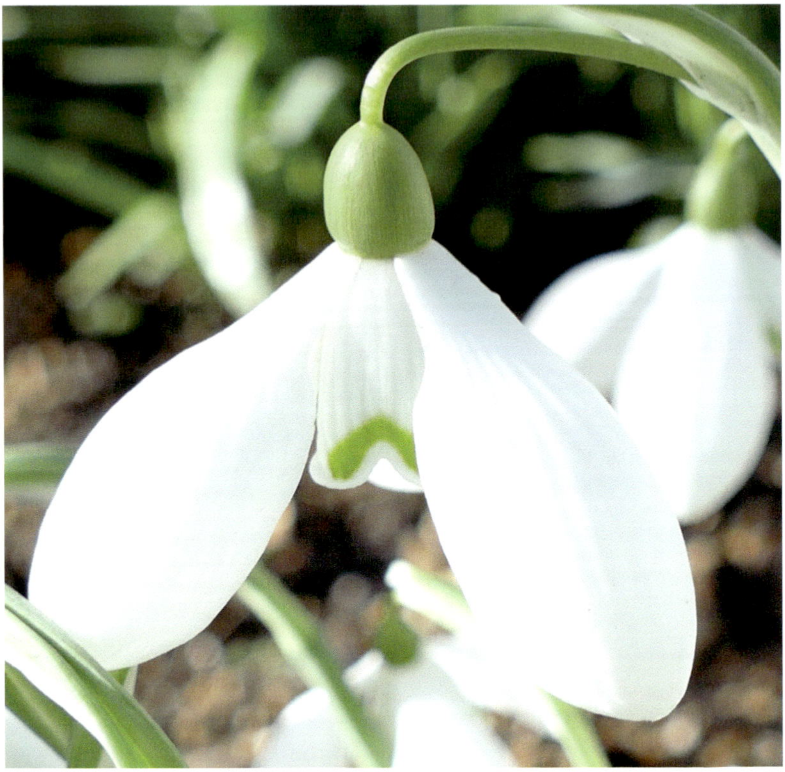

Figure 68 'Mighty Atom'.

mid-later flowering snowdrops, and both are smaller, so-called dumpy snowdrops, flowering close to the soil. 'Tubby Merlin', like 'Merlin', has an almost complete green inner marking on the inner perianth segments. Named in the 1960s, 'Tubby Merlin' is still regarded as a good snowdrop, clumping up well. 'Anne of Geierstein' is another latish, smallish snowdrop, just emerging with large flowers, said to be quite rare (Figure 10). It is an attractive old variety but is not quick to form a clump. I have had it for over 8 years and have not yet felt able to divide it.

Let me get back to the 'Rodmarton' snowdrops – selected by Simon Biddulph of Rodmarton Manor, Gloucestershire. 'Rodmarton Sirius' (Figure 48) is a medium height snowdrop with very distinctive inner flower markings and an olive-green ovary, characteristic of the slender snowdrop, *G. gracilis*. 'Rodmarton Capella' (Figure 49), on the other hand, is a much taller snowdrop with broad leaves and very dark green inner flower markings, although not as tall as 'Rodmarton Regulus'. Although these Rodmarton snowdrops emerged earlier, they are fully out now and are looking good.

Plants just coming now are 'Lavinia' – the last of my Greatorex double hybrids to come into flower, but still very welcome for its neat appearance. The well-known 'Pusey Green Tips' double is now flowering. It is another, rather diminutive 'Flore Pleno'-type double with distorted inner florets but, as its name suggests, selected because of the obvious green tips on the outer florets. It is thought to have originated from the village of Pusey, Oxfordshire in 1938.

21 FEBRUARY

All the snowdrops in my garden are now flowering. We have had some warmish weather over the last few days with some sunshine. The last few snowdrops to flower have responded to this. So much for snowdrops emerging in March. Perhaps in cooler parts of the UK, snowdrops would still wait for March or even April to emerge.

First let me mention some snowdrop species. So far virtually all the snowdrops described from my garden have been species, subspecies, varieties or hybrids of *G. reginae-olgae, G. elwesii*, *G. nivalis*, *G. plicatus* or *G. gracilis*. But taxonomists have recognized 22 different species of snowdrops (see Chapter One, Table 1). I grow two more of these 22 species snowdrops that come out late.

One, Woronow's snowdrop (*G. woronowii*), has quite small unassuming flowers, but compensates by having attractive, bright green foliage, very obviously different from most flowering snowdrops (Figure 33). Woronow's snowdrop clumps up well and can be divided frequently. I have both a shorter and longer-leaved variety, and also another variety which has more matt leaves and double green markings on the inner petals.

Another late-flowering species, the alpine snowdrop, *G. alpinus,* is more interesting than Woronow's snowdrop because it is rarer in cultivation and has largish flowers on a rather short plant. It is said to clump up slowly, but my clone seems to be doing fine.

A classic late snowdrop, 'Allenii', noted for its strong scent supposedly of bitter almonds, is in flower (Figure 9). It is a very old snowdrop named in honour of James Allen in 1891, and formerly thought to be a hybrid. But DNA sequence evidence now suggests it is a variant of *G. alpinus*.[66] It has quite wide leaves, short and spreading at the time of flowering, with an attractive flower. It is slow to clump up. My clump has produced only 10 offsets in over 10 years.

Two more yellow snowdrops, 'Primrose Warburg' (Figure 69) and 'Lady Elphinstone' (Figure 70), a double, are in flower. They are slightly later than the other yellows, 'Wendy's Gold' and 'Spindlestone Surprise'. Some say that 'Primrose Warburg' should be merged with 'Spindlestone Surprise', i.e. that they are the same variety. But the fact that I grow them side by side and one always flowers later than the other suggests they are distinct clones. 'Primrose Warburg' was collected from the late Primrose Warburg's Oxford garden and named after her in 1997. 'Lady Elphinstone' is an old yellow snowdrop, very similar to 'Flore Pleno' but with yellow markings instead of green, found in Heawood Hall, Cheshire, and named in 1890. It is said to be difficult to grow and variable with the markings (green rather than yellow) in some years. But, so far, my clump of 'Lady Elphinstone' has come up year after year, keeping its yellow markings.

I do not grow the recently introduced, very fashionable and expensive yellow snowdrop, 'Elizabeth Harrison', or the newest orange snowdrops, 'Anglesey Orange Tip', but I do grow a half-yellow 'Blonde Inge', which is flowering now and has clumped up well (Figure 71). Discovered in Germany in 1977, this is a fairly small, common snowdrop-type cultivar that has a normal green ovary, but when the flower opens it reveals a yellow marking on the inner flower, although in some flowers it is green. In other words, it is variable. Another common snowdrop-type cultivar, 'Elfin', found in 1997, is also in flower. This snowdrop is characterized by its small size and green tips on the flowers.

The famous snowdrop, 'Trym', named after the village Westbury on Trym, near Bristol where it was found in the late 1980s, is now flowering. Unusually, the outer flower petals are short and boldly marked in green, closely resembling the inner ones. When mature the outer segments of the flower curl out resembling the eaves of a Chinese

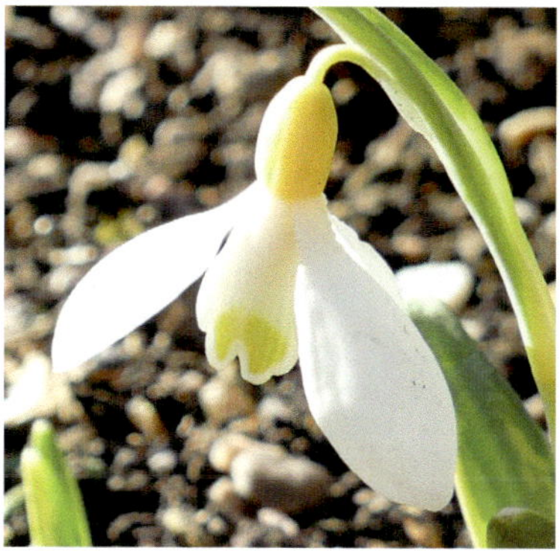

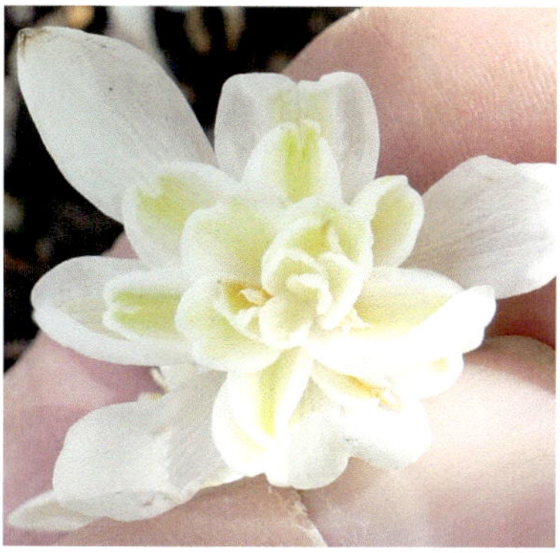

[Left] Figure 69 'Primrose Warburg'.

[Right] Figure 70 'Lady Elphinstone'.

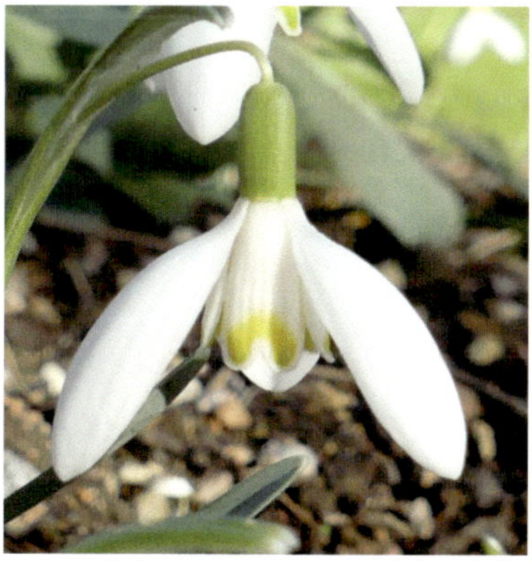

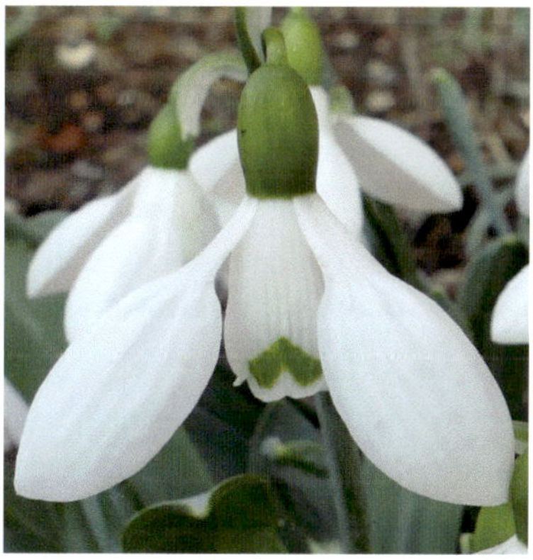

[Left] Figure 71 'Blonde Inge'.

[Right] Figure 72 'Mandarin'.

pagoda. 'Trym' is a strong snowdrop that bulks up well, and is the parent of the earlier flowering seedling, 'Trimmer', already mentioned. Joe Sharman, the famous galanthophile, crossed 'Trym' with another yellow Crimean-type snowdrop to produce 'Golden Fleece'. A single bulb sold for £1,390 on Ebay in 2015 which was then a world record price for one bulb!

'Mandarin' (Figure 72) is another robust snowdrop with an olive-green ovary that has been flowering for some time but is looking

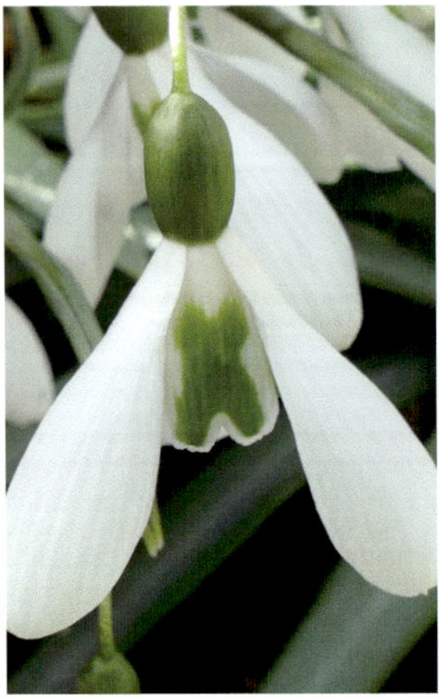

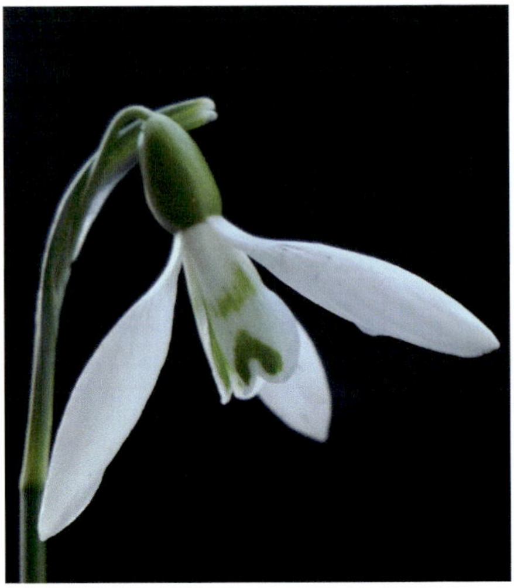

[Left] Figure 73 'Sally Ann'.

[Right] Figure 74 'David Shackleton'.

particularly good now. Found in a garden in Longlevens, Gloucestershire in the 1990s and named for its oriental-like appearance, it is a very bold snowdrop with wide leaves.

'Greenfields' is another late snowdrop that is just emerging. It is an older Irish snowdrop from the 1950s of quite short stature. This is a good late snowdrop to grow, as it bulks up well in a relatively short time. Two other late snowdrops of distinction are now flowering. 'Sally Ann', named in the late 1950s after the daughter of Herbert Ransom, has good inner flower markings with a thick green cross (Figure 73). 'Peg Sharples' is a bit later and is widely grown for its late-flowering habit and attractive flowers with good markings. It was raised from seed by Peg Sharples in Cumbria in the 1960s.

I also grow 'David Shackleton' – another late snowdrop, known since the 1960s – named after an Irish plantsman (Figure 74). It shows off its rather pointed flowers well clear of the shorter upright leaves. Another late snowdrop, 'Bill Bishop', named in 1998 after the plantsman at Harrogate, Yorkshire, has truly enormous flowers, as does the aptly named 'Miller's Late' that flowers quite close to the ground. 'Miller's Late' has wide leaves and a well-developed arching spathe, but who the

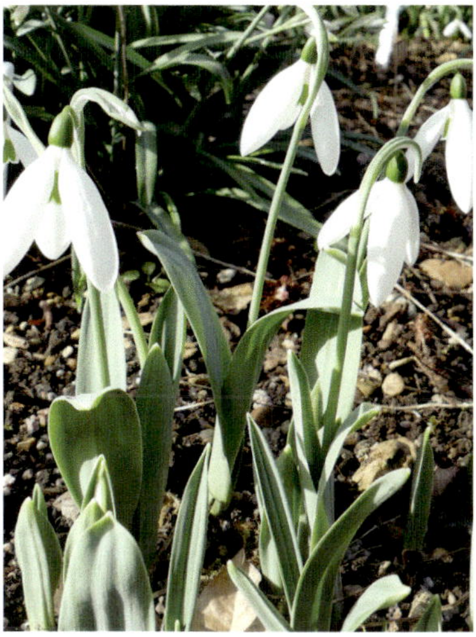

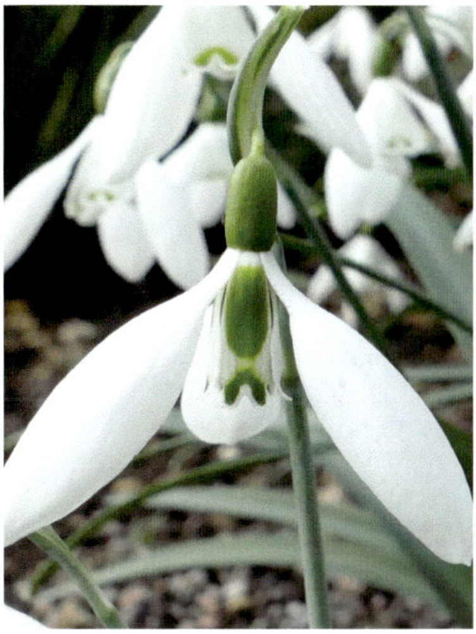

[Left] Figure 75 'Miller's Late'.

[Right] Figure 76 'St Anne's'.

Miller was is unknown (Figure 75). 'Peg Sharples', 'David Shackleton', 'Bill Bishop' and 'Miller's Late' are all rather short plants at the time of flowering, but no less attractive for that. These four varieties should be planted at the front of a border so they can easily be admired.

I have another snowdrop called 'St Anne's' that comes out late. I like this snowdrop a lot (Figure 76). I had to buy it again because I lost it recently. Needless to say, I have replanted it in a different position to exclude the possibility that infection caused its demise. 'St Anne's' is a very upright snowdrop, with pointed rather than rounded outer flower segments and good inner markings. It is named after St Anne's Manor, Sutton Bonnington, Nottingham, once the home of Barbara Buchanan.

Another latish snowdrop is the Crimean snowdrop species, *G. plicatus*. I have two different clones bought from different sources. They are principally noteworthy because of their broad leaves with upturned (plicate) margins, which is also seen in many of the *G. plicatus* hybrids, e.g. 'Wendy's Gold'. But the flowers, at least in my clones, are unremarkable. They do not clump up well, so I would not particularly recommend them.

5 MARCH

The snowdrop season is coming to an end, but the late snowdrops are still looking good, and the yellows are still attractive. 'Trym' is looking good, as is 'Mandarin', 'Greenfields', 'Anne of Geierstein' and 'Miller's Late'. 'Bill Bishop', 'Peg Sharples', 'Sally Ann' and 'Merlin' are still very attractive. Amongst the doubles, 'Blewbury Tart', 'Cordelia', 'Jaquenetta', 'Lavinia', 'Rodmarton' and 'Pusey Green Tips' are still flowering. The yellow 'Spindlestone Surprise', 'Primrose Warburg' and the late double 'Lady Elphinstone' are still looking good, although 'Wendy's Gold' has finished flowering now. We must not forget the species snowdrop, Woronow's snowdrop (*G. woronowii*), which is now at its best (Figure 33). It is among the latest of the snowdrops to flower. I must also not forget the common snowdrop, *G. nivalis,* and the double form 'Flore Pleno' (Figure 17), both of which are still flowering. If my garden were in a colder zone, such as in the north of England or up in the Cotswolds, I would expect more snowdrops to be still out now.

Have any snowdrops failed to flower this year? Yes, I have two separate clumps of the double 'Titania'. Although plenty leaves were present, neither has flowered. 'Edith' also failed to flower this year. My clumps of 'Diggory' and 'Scharlockii' look weaker and had fewer flowers than last year. All these varieties need moving and splitting to encourage flowers next year.

The last two weeks have given me the opportunity to buy 'replacement' snowdrops – varieties that I have lost. I have repurchased 'Hill Poë' – a famous Irish double snowdrop, described over 100 years ago, but one that I have yet to find a good position to establish it in my garden. 'Hill Poë' is quite diminutive and is easily lost in my experience. I have also added 'South Hayes' and 'Green Necklace' to my collection. 'South Hayes' is a much sought-after snowdrop, named in honour of the late Primrose Warburg's Oxford garden, where it was discovered in the early 1990s, probably as a seedling of 'Trym'. It is not unlike 'Trym'. There is an 'exclamation-like' green mark on its outer flower segment that differs from 'Trym' and 'Trimmer', which only has a single mark. 'Green Necklace' is a common snowdrop (*G. nivalis*) variant found by Daphne Chappell in Ruth Birchall's garden in the 1970s and is noted for its inner flower markings reminiscent of a necklace. I bought it at the late

Ruth Birchall's garden, Cotswold Farm, Gloucestershire. That is the fun of growing snowdrops. There are always new varieties you would like in your garden, assuming you have space and can finance them.

I should mention the snowflakes (*Leucojum*), which are related to the snowdrops but differ in having their six floral segments of equal length. The snowflakes often have multiple flowers grouped together, rather than a solitary flower, as in the snowdrops. I grow the spring snowflake, *Leucojum vernum,* and the Easter snowflake, *Leucojum aestivum*. Both are easy to grow and complement snowdrops well. The spring snowflake (*L. vernum*) is about the same size as the larger snowdrops and flowers in February, but the Easter snowflake (*L. aestivum*) is later and taller and is now in flower.

13 March

After some fine weather over the last few days the snowdrop season is really ending. Only Woronow's snowdrop (*G. woronowii*), 'Miller's Late' and 'Peg Sharples' have unfaded flowers, enough to bring into the house as a posy. The emphasis is changing in the garden, with the aconites, the early daffodils, colourful crocuses and early apricot and cherry blossom out. There are even a few butterflies to be seen in the warm afternoon sunshine. The snowdrops are still growing, their leaves extending in length and the seed heads forming, except for the doubles, which are infertile. I do not cut off the seed heads, and rather let them seed around. There is evidence of seedlings growing around several different clumps in my garden.

16 March

Out of interest, I measured the length of some of my snowdrop leaves today. The longest, 48 cm and 3 cm at its broadest point, was *G. plicatus* ssp. *plicatus.* Many snowdrops had leaves longer than 30 cm, including 'Regulus', 'Comet', 'Magnet', 'Florence Baker' and 'Atkinsii'. 'Comet' and 'Florence Baker' had the widest leaves – as much as 3.5 cm at their broadest point. Most snowdrop leaves arch upwards and outwards, but some are noticeably spread out at soil level, such as Queen Olga's snowdrop (*G. reginae-olgae*).

31 MARCH

All my snowdrops have now finished flowering, although the Easter snowflake, *L. aestivum*, is still looking good. This is the best time to transplant snowdrops in the green, or to swap snowdrops as I usually have more bulbs than I need when splitting up clumps.

I have given or swapped snowdrops with many fellow galanthophiles over the years, and this is the ideal way to get to know other gardeners. These include Simon Bagnall, head of gardens and grounds at Worcester College, Oxford; Susan Kasper at St Edmund Hall, Oxford; and the gardener at my own college, Lincoln College, Oxford. These gardens, other Oxford college gardens and also the Oxford Botanic Garden – the first ever botanic garden in the UK that was founded in 1621 as a 'physic' garden – are open to the public and are definitely worth visiting in February and March to admire their snowdrops.

I do not know when the first snowdrop was grown in these Oxford gardens. St Edmund Hall is thought to be built on land occupied by an Edmund of Abingdon in the early fourteenth century.[67] Worcester College, formerly Gloucester College, stands on the site of a Benedictine monastery,[68] and so it is possible the common snowdrop, imported by monks from Europe, grew there much earlier than we know from written sources.[69]

Six

SNOWDROP ART

Photographic or painted images of snowdrops abound and are popular on greetings cards, Christmas cards and almost anywhere one looks. Why is this? I suspect it is the beauty and simplicity of the predominantly white flower with its image of purity that appeals to most people. The snowdrop is also one of the first plants to flower in the year and is admired as a herald of approaching spring and better weather.

The name snowdrop is not that old and was first published in Gerard's impressive English herbal in 1633,[70] although the word was definitely in use earlier in 1615, albeit with a slightly different spelling.[71] The English word, snowdrop, may be derived from the German 'Schneetropfen' (literally, snow drop), which refers to the earrings or pendants worn in the sixteenth and seventeenth centuries. The even older English names for snowdrops are thought to be Candlemas Bells, Fair Maid of February or White Ladies – names all connected with the Christian festival of Candlemas Day.[72] This may refer to the procession of white-robed maidens that took place on the 'Feast of the Purification' on 2 February.

The first unambiguous image of the common snowdrop, *G. nivalis*, in early publications was a woodcut in a European sixteenth century herbal by Dodoens (Figure 77) in 1568.[73] He named it *Leucoion bulb. triphyllon*, which can be translated as 'white bulbous three-petalled flower'. This same woodcut – reused[74] – was reproduced in many other later sixteenth and early seventeenth century herbals, including those

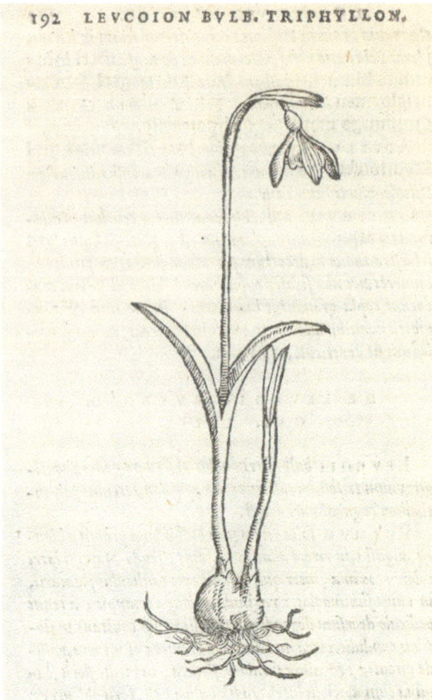

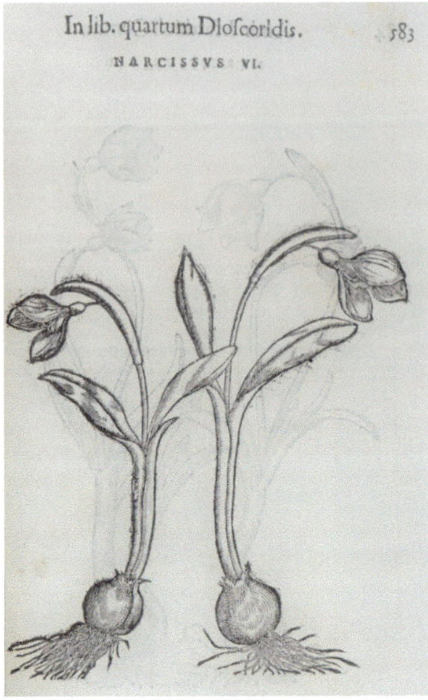

[Left] Figure 77 *Leucoion bulb. triphyllon* (common snowdrop, *G. nivalis*), from Dodoens, 1568 (© The Bodleian Library, University of Oxford, page 192).

[Right] Figure 78 *Narcissus* (common snowdrop, *G. nivalis*), from Matthioli, 1583 (© The President and Fellows of Magdalen College, Oxford).

of L'Obel,[75] L'Ecluse (Clusius),[76] and Gerard[77] in English. Confusingly, many different names were used in these herbals for the same snowdrop image.

The woodcut reproduced in Figure 77, which included the bulb and roots, cannot be considered a work of art but was sufficiently accurate to allow easy identification along with the descriptions in the text. It is true that Matthioli[78], in 1554, had published a woodcut, labelled '*Narcissus*' with the flower of a snowdrop but the bulb and leaves of a daffodil. This 'hybrid' looks very odd, but perhaps his illustrator had picked a snowdrop flower, without the leaves and the bulb, and had assumed it was a new type of daffodil. Later, in 1583, a posthumous publication by Matthioli[79] included a correct woodcut of a snowdrop, although it was still named *Narcissus* (Figure 78).

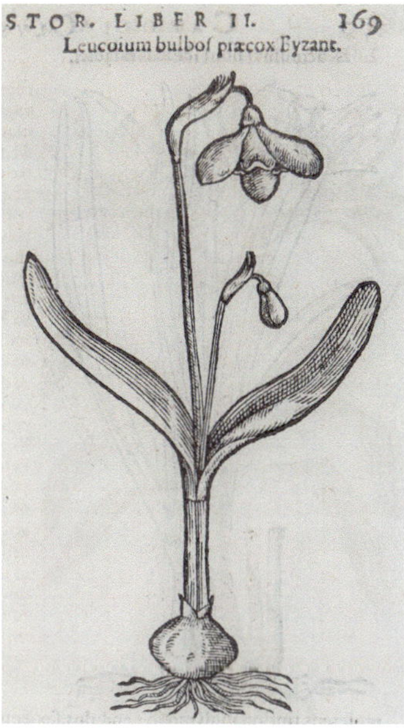

Figure 79 *Leucoion bulbos. praecox Byzant.* (Crimean snowdrop, *G. plicatus*), from L'Ecluse, 1601 (© The President and Fellows of Magdalen College, Oxford).

The more robust snowdrop, the Crimean snowdrop, *G. plicatus*, originally from Byzantium (modern-day Istanbul), was not recognized as a different plant from the common snowdrop until 1583 – in an early herbal by L'Ecluse.[80] However, it was not illustrated until 1601 (Figure 79) in his later work.[81] The magnificent early sixteenth century European herbals of Brunfels[82] in 1536 and Fuchs[83] in 1542 do not mention snowdrops, but in Fuchs there is a beautiful hand-coloured image of a snowflake, labelled *Viola alba*. Apparently, snowflakes (*L. vernum*) were better known, or more highly valued than snowdrops in the early sixteenth century.

These early herbals were designed to be hand-coloured after printing, although most herbals I have examined were uncoloured. Despite the lack of colouring, many herbals were published in numerous editions and languages and sold in their tens of thousands.[84,85]

We must remember that the explosion in interest in herbals was not primarily for readers to admire the plants or their flowers. These herbals were the medical texts of the sixteenth and seventeenth centuries used by physicians to identify plants accurately for their use in medicine to treat common ailments, such as pain, toothache, use in childbirth, indigestion, headache, vomiting, diarrhoea, etc. Dodoens[86] even recommends a diet of quinces, saying that pregnant women 'who often eat quinces will bring forth wise children of good understanding'. Nevertheless, snowdrops had no known medical use then, so they and some other plants, were included for their intrinsic interest, or perhaps

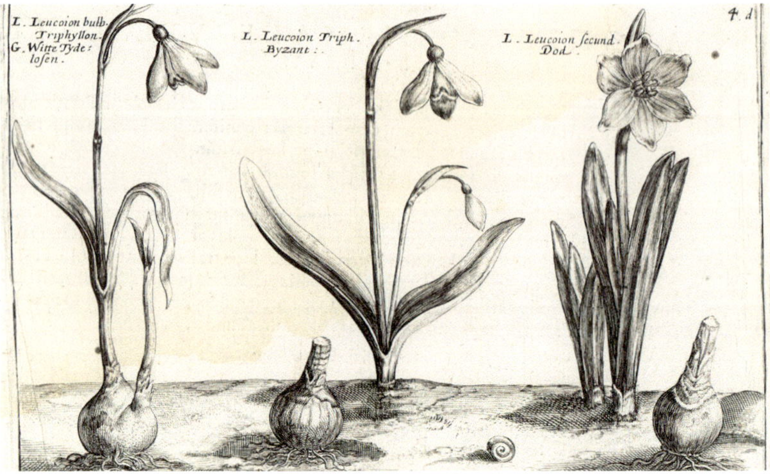

Figure 80 *Leucoion bulb. Triphyllon* (common snowdrop, *G. nivalis*, left), and *Leucoion Triphyllon Byzant.* (Crimean snowdrop, *G. plicatus) and Leucoion Secund. Dod.* (*Narcissus* sp., right) from de Passe, 1614 *Hortus Floridus* (with permission, Sherardian Library, one of the Bodleian Libraries of the University of Oxford).

because the authors realized they might be useful for medicine in the future.

In the seventeenth century, woodcuts were starting to go out of fashion as metal plate engraving showed more detail of the plants than could easily be achieved in woodcuts. An impressive 1614 herbal by de Passe[87] uses metal plate engraving to illustrate *G. nivalis* and *G. plicatus,* alongside a daffodil (Figure 80). De Passe is admired for his naturalism and botanical accuracy as an engraver. The plate is a miniature landscape as the plants are shown growing in soil at the artist's eye level, giving the impression that the flowers are standing up from the landscape. De Passe embellishes the landscape with a small snail, whilst in other plates he includes a bee, a rabbit or a mouse.

Besler's[88] *Hortus Eystettensis* (1613) also used the newer metal plate engraving to illustrate plants. In Besler, botanical accuracy was definitely secondary to a decorative, if rather stylized, effect that was enhanced by the impressive elephant folio size of the prints. Calligraphy was important and often letters were intermingled with

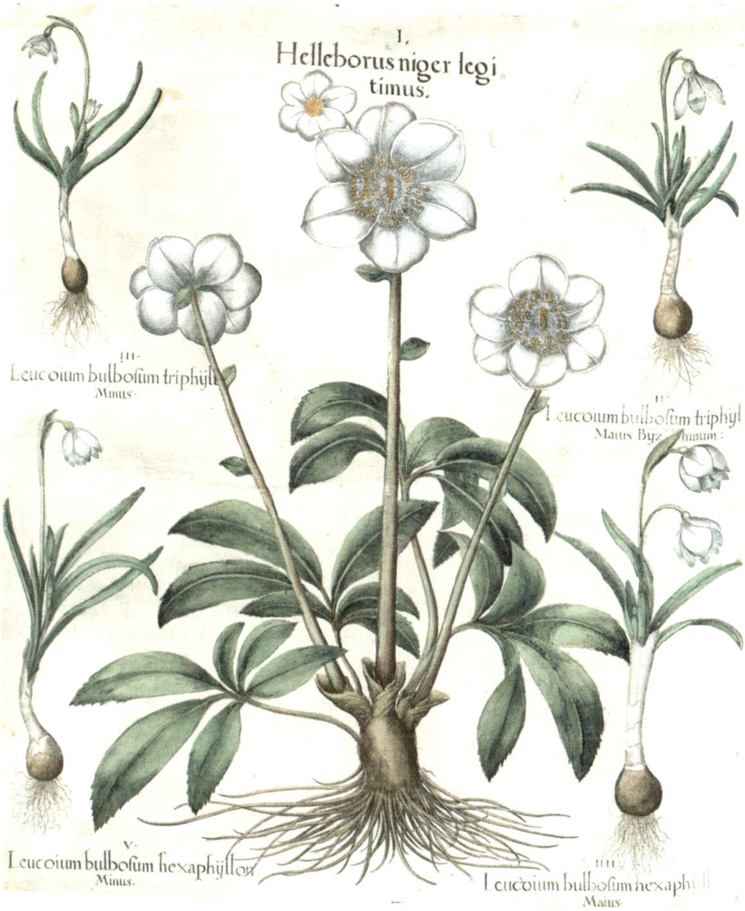

Figure 81 Christmas rose surrounded by snowdrops and snowflakes, from Besler, 1613, *Hortus Eystettensis*, plate 361, shelf number 183/1 SJ II 2894–3, University Library, Eichstätt-Ingolstadt, Germany (with permission).

the lines of the plants. Roots were very amply illustrated and became part of the decorative effect. Figure 81 lavishly illustrates a rather upright and formalized Christmas rose *(Helleborus niger)* that takes centre stage. Snowdrops, along with snowflakes, are almost incidental, tucked away in the corners. Scale is unimportant because the common snowdrop *G. nivalis* (top left) is shown almost as large as the larger Crimean snowdrop *G. plicatus* (top right). The two snowflakes, the

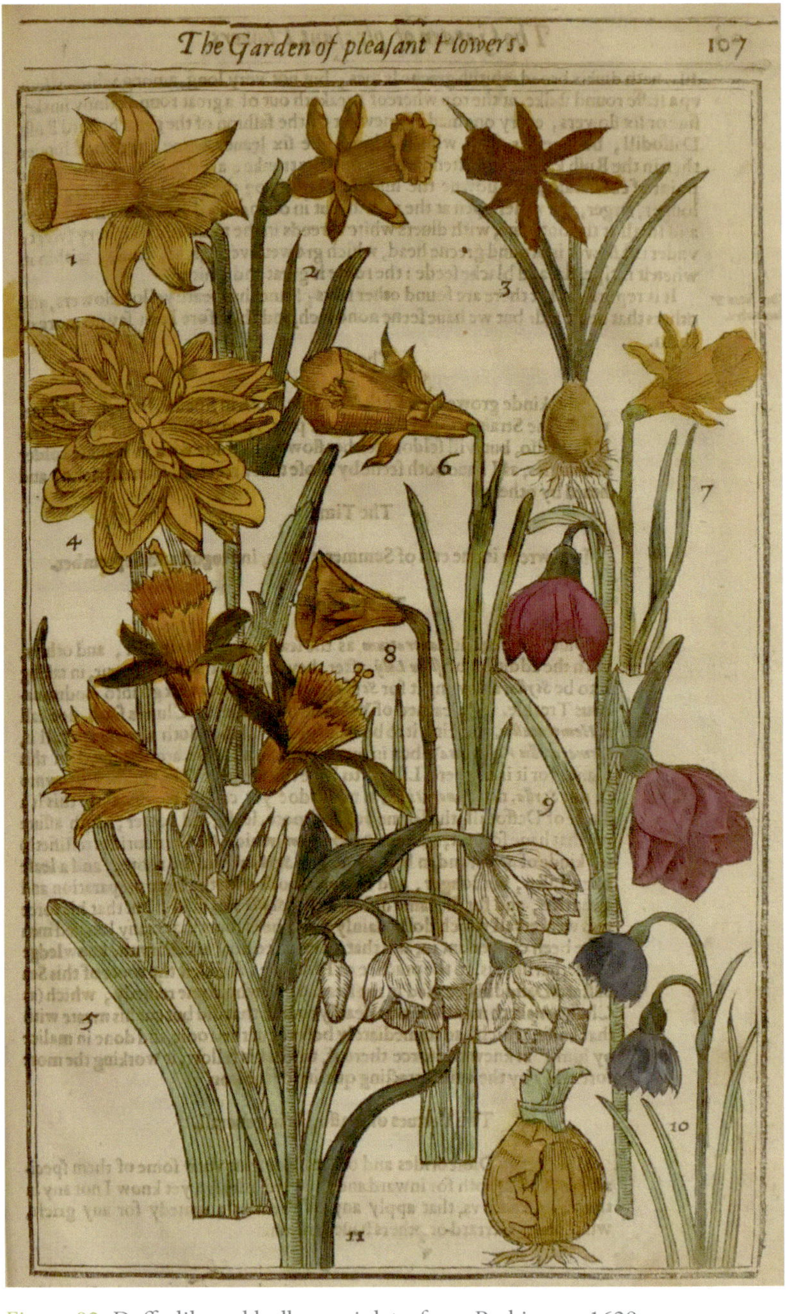

Figure 82 Daffodils and bulbous violets, from Parkinson, 1629.

spring snowflake, *L. vernum* (bottom left) and the Easter snowflake, *L. aestivum* (bottom right) should be almost twice as tall as the *Galanthus* species but are shown at similar size. No matter; Besler is still a magnificent, very early illustrator of snowdrops even if botanical accuracy is compromised.

Another important early English herbal was John Parkinson's,[89] *Paradisi in Sole Paradisus Terrestris* or '*The garden of pleasant flowers, the kitchen garden and the orchard*', published in 1629. It appeared just before, and in competition with, the much-enlarged Johnson's second edition (1633) of Gerard's herbal. In Parkinson, as in Besler before him, the illustrations of plants are arranged in groups in a tabloid format, rather than individually as in Gerard, usually occupying a whole page in groups of up to 10 or more different plants. This tabloid format of Parkinson is artistically more pleasing than Gerard's and the earlier herbals of the sixteenth century, but some botanical detail is lost (Figure 82). Surprisingly, the common snowdrop (*G. nivalis*) and the Crimean snowdrop (*G. plicatus*) are clearly described in Parkinson as bulbous violets, i.e. the lesser early bulbous violet and the Byzantine lesser early bulbous violet, but they are not illustrated. However, snowflakes are illustrated in the figure – although the flowers of *L. vernum,* are incorrectly coloured reddish-violet. This error is perhaps excusable because of the English name in use at the time – 'the great early bulbous violet' – although the description in the text clearly states it has a white flower. Perhaps the person doing the colouring was not shown the text! The Johnson (1633) edition of Gerard, however, illustrated both the common (Figure 2) and Crimean (or Byzantine) (Figure 3) snowdrops, reusing the woodcuts from the Plantin workshop, as can be seen by comparing Figure 77 with Figure 2 and Figure 79 with Figure 3.

The illustrations in the later floral publications of the eighteenth and nineteenth century seem to be of two types. There were those that were aimed at a more general audience, where the artistry of the images was more important than botanical accuracy, and there were those published for botanists, who were interested in classifying species and who wanted more botanical detail.

Thornton's *Temple of Flora*,[90] published in the early 1800s, takes botanical art further into the realm of the exotic. The drawings are more accurate than in Besler, but the botanical value is still limited. Yet Thornton is admired for the artistry of the images. His idea was to have plants drawn in a natural and usually idyllic landscape – a style of painting that had not been widely practised before in plant illustrations, although it had been anticipated to some extent by de Passe with his miniature landscapes almost two centuries before.[91] It is surprising that Thornton, who illustrated a mere 31 plants, decided to include snowdrops in one of his plates (Figure 83), as this mezzotint must be the least showy and least exotic of all his plates. Perhaps it was included because it was the only image to show a wintry, snowy landscape, possibly also a night-time painting lit up by moonlight. It strongly contrasts with all other plates in the *Temple of Flora*, including the more famous images of carnations and tulips.

While Besler's and Thornton's publications were not generally available to botanists or those interested in botanical art because of their extremely high price, Anne Pratt's[92] *Flowering Plants of Great Britain* was a popular mid-Victorian publication. She wanted her flora to be used by those 'who had not hitherto studied Botany' and drew all the images herself, collaborating with William Dickes for the printing. Moreover, in her introduction, she states that she uses 'English, rather than Latin, so as to adapt the *Flora* to the use of the unscientific'. Her descriptions are very informative and readable, the images very pleasing artistically, and reasonably accurate botanically. She groups snowdrops together with snowflakes and daffodils, in an artistic way, although the colouring of the common snowdrop (Figure 84) shows yellowing in the petals, which anticipates 'yellow' snowdrops by quite a few years! This incorrect colouring of the common snowdrop is attributed to imperfections in the chromolithographic process of preparing images, which sometimes led to mistakes in colouring.

Another popular series in late Victorian England aimed at the general reader was Hulme's[93] *Familiar wild flowers* in five volumes. Hulme was art master at Marlborough College and was responsible for the drawings. Figure 85 shows a lithograph of snowdrops with a snowflake. Although a pleasing composition, the shading of the petals, while giving more depth to the image, somewhat dulls the white flowers. Hulme obviously liked strong shading. He also included

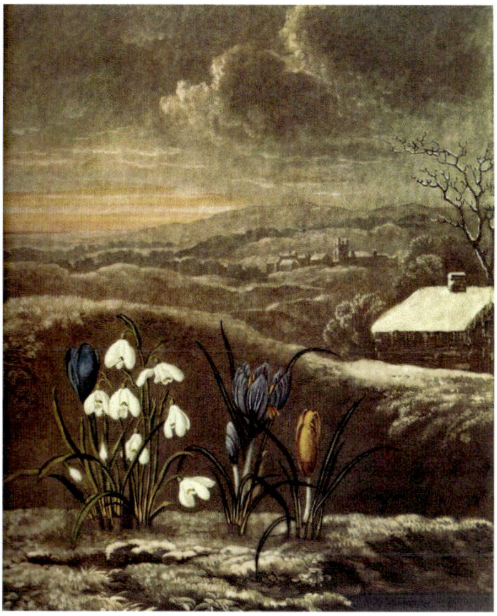

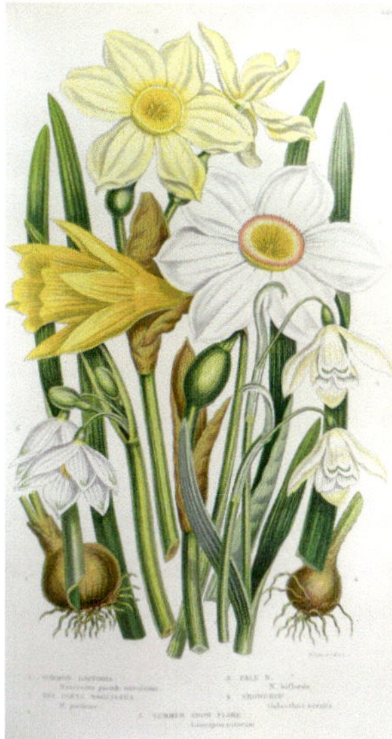

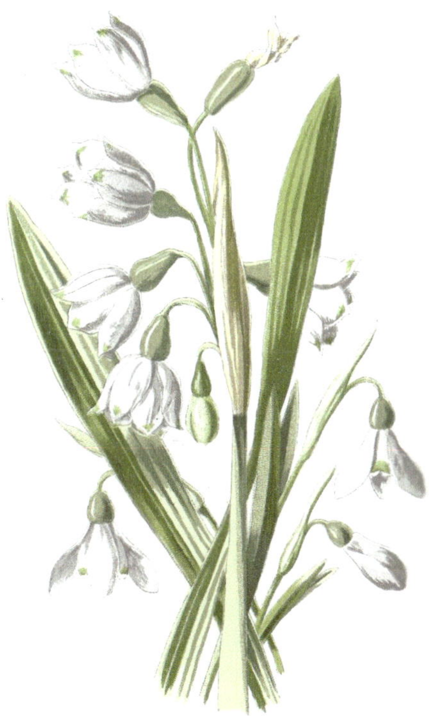

[Upper Left] Figure 83 The snowdrop, from Thornton, *Temple of Flora,* 1804, plate IV.

[Upper Right] Figure 84 Daffodils, snowdrops and snowflake, from Pratt, 1873, vol. 5, plate 220.

[Left] Figure 85 Snowdrops (*G. nivalis*) and snowflake (*L. aestivum*), from Hulme, 1875–1900.

vignettes, with a range of different styles of background shading, in his description of the snowdrop.

Development of botanically accurate images of flowers, including the snowdrop, that showed details of the flower structure was really only developed in the late eighteenth century by James Sowerby[94] in his 36-volume treatise *English Botany* published between 1790–1814. The naming of plants followed the then relatively new, binomial, sexual system of classification of plants by Linnaeus. The descriptions and accompanying hand-coloured engravings are of exceptional quality. James Sowerby, a trained botanical artist, worked with James Edward Smith, who wrote almost all the accompanying descriptions, and established a successful collaboration between an artist and botanist. All 2,592 prints were based on original drawings by Sowerby – drawn over a 23-year period.

The common snowdrop (*G. nivalis*) had pride of place in volume 1 of Sowerby published in 1790. Plate 19 showed not only an accurate representation of the snowdrop, but also included four small additions (Figure 86, bottom left of the image) that showed individual parts – the ovary, style and stamens within the flower. The accompanying description is written with the general reader in mind and tells us 'No plant is more generally cultivated, or more cordially welcome as the herald of approaching spring.' Sowerby did not group related plants together, as Gerard and Parkinson had done almost 200 years earlier. But the great skill of Sowerby was his artistry and botanical accuracy, which greatly surpassed most earlier publications.

Sowerby's *English Botany* was stimulated by William Curtis,[95] who three years earlier in 1787 had started a periodical *The Botanical Magazine*. It was aimed at 'Ladies, Gentlemen and Gardeners, as wish to become scientifically acquainted with the plants they cultivate.' It was a highly successful publication mainly because of its exquisite hand-coloured plates and the fact that it included flowers from all over the world. It is still published today – now online. Curtis employed Sowerby, who contributed many plates in the first four volumes,[96] which he usually signed. But we do not know if he, or another painter, drew the unsigned spring snowflake (*L. vernum*) illustrated in volume 2 in 1788 (Figure 87). It was not until later, in 1820, that the Crimean

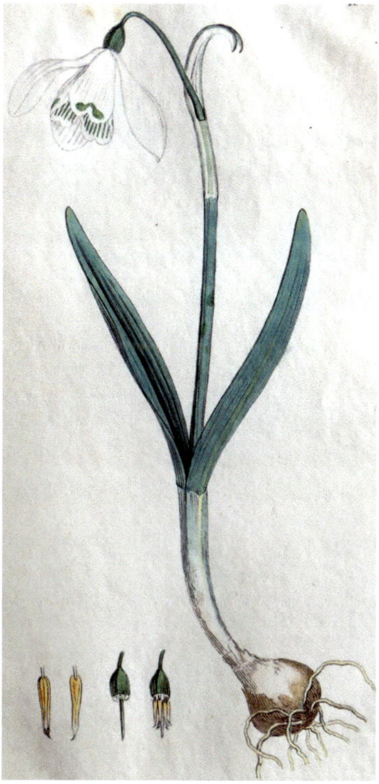

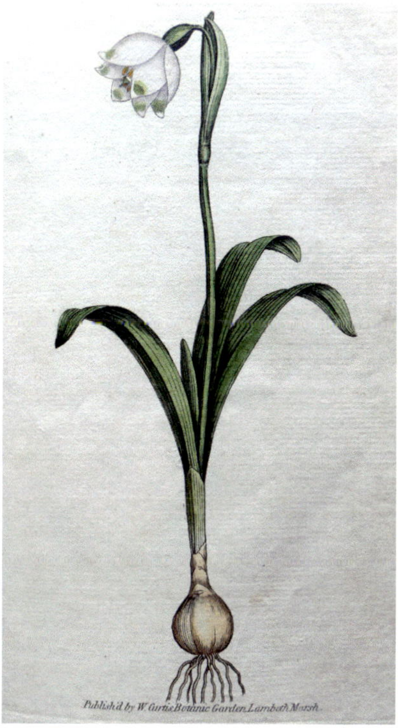

[Left] Figure 86 Common snowdrop (*G. nivalis*), from Sowerby, 1790, vol. 1.

[Right] Figure 87 Spring snowflake (*L. vernum*), Curtis, 1788, vol. 2.

snowdrop (*G. plicatus*) was illustrated in Curtis, albeit incorrectly drawn with four leaves.

Other publications which explored more systematically the flora of the UK emerged in the early nineteenth century, e.g. William Baxter's 'British flowering plants' or, more correctly, *British Phaenogamous Botany* in six volumes from 1834.[97] This work was aimed at students of botany, but still retained high-quality hand-coloured plates. Costs were reduced by showing figures for only one species in a given genus. Baxter, who was curator of Oxford Botanic Garden, has more detailed descriptions of plants than Curtis or Sowerby. This work thus anticipates the floras that emerged later in the nineteenth and twentieth century. The common snowdrop (*G. nivalis*) (Figure 88) was included in volume 1.

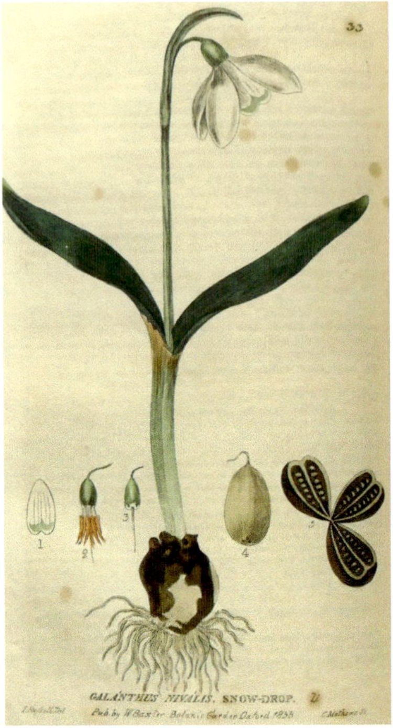

Figure 88 Common snowdrop (*G. nivalis*), Baxter, 1834, vol. 1.

This image is considered to be superior to Sowerby's because Baxter included, in his inserts, clearer images of the dissected flower structure, the capsule and seeds.

In the late nineteenth century and the twentieth century, botanical floras appeared – such as Clapham, Tutin and Warburg's *Flora of the British Isles* in 1958[98] but without illustrations. A detailed 'key' was included so that the keen amateur botanist could theoretically identify any flowering plant from scratch – with the aid of a ×10 magnifying lens. However, there was a need for illustrations. A companion volume of simple black and white line drawings,[99] more like sketches, duly appeared, which helped a bit.

In the last 50 years, I think there has been a reaction to the former strictly botanical approach of describing plants, necessary though this is for the taxonomist. The distinction has always been blurred between what the early herbalists or botanist wanted, and those who were not trained botanists but were interested in learning about plants. The public wanted to know more about flowers they might come across when walking in the countryside or which flowers to grow in their gardens. Even in Gerard's time, snowdrops were included – not because they were useful (they had no known value as a medicine then), but because '*they are maintained and cherished in gardens for the beautie and rarenesse of the floures, and sweetnesse of their smell*'.

One might think that modern floras might be filled with photographic images of plants given the ease of digital photography.

In general, this has not happened. Blamey,[100] for instance, following the publication of her successful earlier *Mediterranean Flora*, produced in 2003 a comprehensive British and Irish flora with over 5,000 illustrations of hand-painted wildflowers where the flowers are arranged in groups of 10 or more per page that are integral to the flora. These coloured drawings help identification immensely. Descriptions are minimal – to keep the book within reasonable length – but are usually enough to identify the plant. As a botanical artist, Blamey has a huge advantage over a photographer in that small additions can be included – just as Sowerby did two centuries earlier – showing details of flower structure or showing images of fruits to aid identification. However, the snowdrop images in Blamey are not particularly well drawn, possibly because of space limitations.

Flowers have been painted in watercolours throughout history, but I have not attempted to show any snowdrop paintings because such images are not generally accessible, except on websites. Many other art forms have been used to display flowers, such as the glass flowers by Blaschka in the Ware Collection in Harvard University, USA. Unfortunately this extensive and exquisite collection of over 830 plant species does not include snowdrops. However, interesting abstract images of snowdrops were painted on ceramic tiles and used to decorate Victorian and Edwardian homes, such as the art nouveau Stoke pottery example in Figure 89. This may have been used as one of a series of snowdrop tiles surrounding a fireplace.

In summary, this historical survey of the development of snowdrop illustrations over five centuries has shown the range of techniques and styles used. Today's botanical artists[101] usually elect to use watercolours because of the shades of interpretation and subtlety of colour possible with this medium. However, watercolours present particular difficulties when painting the predominantly white flowers of snowdrops. The major difficulty is preventing the blooms from looking grey. The lack of contrast with the white background of watercolour paper also means it is difficult to get the blooms to stand out in a lifelike way, which can be frustrating if the artist is aiming to represent what they see in the garden – little white jewels suspended from the plant like dainty drop earrings. With oil paints or acrylic paints, this problem can be

Figure 89 Snowdrop ceramic tile, made in Stoke, c. 1900.

overcome by painting in a background first, but it is then more difficult to achieve a 'botanical' look to the painting. The choice of medium to achieve the required effect is something that the artist needs to experiment with. Ultimately it is a matter of individual taste.

Another challenge for the artist is keeping the snowdrop in a suitable condition, as painting outside is not ideal in winter. Painting flowers and foliage involves layering paint which can be a lengthy process and take a few days.[102] One possible solution is to pick the flower stem and some leaves, placing them in a jar of water and draw them at room temperature inside the studio. It will be noticed that the three outer petals move upwards within an hour or so because they are sensitive to temperature. This will reveal the inner flower structure as it would be for a pollinating bee on a warm winter's day. At the end of the drawing or painting session the snowdrops in their jar of water can be placed in a fridge – when the petals will close up – and then be taken out the next day to continue painting. With the 'double' snowdrops, this upward movement is minimal because the multiple inner petals and flower structure already mean they are in an open position. An alternative solution would be to paint a snowdrop that had been planted in a small pot, again using a fridge to preserve the integrity of the flower and avoid fading that occurs within 2–3 days if snowdrops are kept inside at room temperature.

Seven

SNOWDROP INDEX: SPECIES, SUBSPECIES AND CULTIVARS

I list all snowdrop species, subspecies and cultivars mentioned in this book as a convenient checklist for readers. The naming of a few cultivars varies according to different sources, but I base my names on well-recognized authorities.[103] I use the abbreviations: (s) for a single snowdrop, (d) for a double snowdrop and (a) for the Award of Garden Merit, AGM, of the British Royal Horticultural Society (RHS) in their 2020 listing. The RHS have rescinded earlier Award of Merits for some cultivars I grow, e.g. 'Bill Bishop', 'Brenda Troyle', 'Hippolyta', 'Ketton' and 'Warham'. Despite this, these are still good snowdrops to cultivate.

I do not identify a cultivar as a hybrid unless it is known without doubt – as in the Greatorex hybrids – because there has been deliberate cross-fertilization between species. The approximate flowering time of the species is given, e.g. the alpine snowdrop *G. alpinus* Fl 2–3, is February to March.

SPECIES AND SUBSPECIES

G. alpinus or alpine snowdrop	Named by Sosnowski in 1911; originally from Georgia; uncommon in cultivation; glaucous green leaves with one apical mark on inner perianth segments; largish flower on a short plant; from Georgia, Russia, Turkey. Variety, *alpinus*, Fl 2–3, is fertile, distinguished from infertile variety, *bortkewitschianus*.

G. angustifolius	Named in 1951 by Koss from southern Russia; rare in wild (Fl 3–5) and in cultivation; narrow leaved.
G. bursanus	Recently described in 2019 from Turkey; rare in the wild; Fl 10–1; fragrant; related to *G. reginae-olgae* ssp. *reginae-olgae*.
G. cilicicus	Named by J. G. Baker in 1897; from Turkey; rare in wild and cultivation; Fl 11–1; related to *G. peshmenii*.
***G. elwesii (a)* or Elwes' snowdrop**	Common in cultivation, variable, parent of many cultivars; from Turkey and Balkans; described by Hooker in 1875 and named after Henry Elwes but type specimen now recognized as *G. gracilis*. Large plant with broad glaucous leaves and bold inner perianth markings; Fl 11–4; variety *elwesii* has two green marks on inner perianth segments; variety *monostictus* (a) has a single apical mark (Figures 5, 16).
G. fosteri	Named by J. G. Baker in 1889; from Turkey, Syria, Lebanon, Jordan; rare in cultivation; a distinctive snowdrop with broad green leaves; Fl 1–4. Possibly not hardy in UK.
G. gracilis	Slender (or graceful) snowdrop; named in 1891 by the Czech botanist Celakovski; from Greece, the Balkans and Turkey; uncommon in cultivation; leaves narrow and often twisted, like a corkscrew; inner perianth segments typically with two marks but can have one large green mark; Fl 1–5.
G. ikariae	Named by J. G. Baker in 1893; from Greek islands, originally from Ikaria; distinguished from other green, broadleaved snowdrops (e.g. *G. woronowii*) by air spaces in the leaves. Fl 1–4; becoming more common in cultivation.
G. koenenianus	Named in 1994 after Koenen who discovered it in 1988 in Turkey; a small snowdrop with distinctive ribbing on the under surface of leaves; rare in wild and in cultivation. Fl 2–3.
G. krasnovii	Named in 1963 after the Russian scientist Krasnov from Georgia; also known in Turkey; distinctive broad green leaves; inner perianth segment lacks an apical notch; rare in wild and in cultivation; Fl 1–5.

G. lagodechianus	Named in 1947 by the Georgian botanist Kemularia-Nathadze; from Georgia; distinguished by narrow green leaves with a single apical mark on inner perianth segments; rare in cultivation. Fl 1–4.
***G. nivalis (a)* or common snowdrop**	Named by Linnaeus in 1753 but previously described in early herbals, the first illustration in Dodoens, 1568 (Figure 77); widespread in Europe and Turkey; introduced into the UK; Fl 1–4 (Figures 1, 7).
G. panjutinii	Named in 2012 in honour of Panjutin, Russian chemist and botanist; closely related to *G. platyphyllus* and *G. krasnovii;* rare in cultivation; Fl 3–6.
G. peshmenii	Named in 1994 by Davis and Brickell after the Turkish scientist, Peshmen; from the Greek island of Kastellorizo and southern Turkey; autumn flowering, before leaves appear – like *G. reginae-olgae* ssp. *reginae-olgae* – but leaves narrower and longer; rare in the wild and uncommon in cultivation; Fl 10–12.
G. platyphyllus	Named in 1948 by American botanists Traub and Moldenke; a broadleaved species from Russia and Georgia closely related to *G. krasnovii* and *G. panjutinii;* apex of inner perianth segments rounded; rare in cultivation; Fl 3–7.
***G. plicatus (a)* or the Crimean (or Clusius') snowdrop**	Named in 1819 but known to Clusius in1583; common in cultivation; a more robust snowdrop than the common snowdrop (*G. nivalis*), and originally from Byzantium (modern-day Istanbul), *G. plicatus* was not recognized as a different plant until 1583 – in an early herbal by Clusius; not illustrated until 1601 in Clusius' later work (Figure 79). *G. plicatus* is named for its folded or 'plicate' leaves, now correctly termed 'explicative', in which the margins of the leaves are folded back against the underside of the leaf (Figures 5, 7, 41). Subspecies *plicatus* has inner perianth segments with one green mark; subspecies *byzantinus* has two green marks; Fl 12–4.
***G. reginae-olgae* or Queen Olga's snowdrop**	Named in 1876 by the Greek botanist, Orphanides, in honour of Queen Olga of Greece (Figure 34) – grandmother of Prince Philip, Duke of Edinburgh (1921–2021); from Greece and Sicily; autumn flowering without leaves present at flowering; otherwise similar to *G. nivalis*. Subspecies *reginae-olgae*

	(a) flowers without leaves present (Figures 13, 19); Fl 9–12. Subspecies *vernalis* (Figure 35*)* has leaves present at flowering and flowers later; Fl 11–1.
G. rizehensis	From Rize; named by Stern in 1956 (although provisionally described in 1934 by G. P. Baker) after the Black Sea coastal town of Rize in Turkey. Known from Georgia, Russia and Turkey; narrow green leaves with a single apical green mark on inner perianth segments; similar to *G. lagodechianus*; uncommon in cultivation; seeds easily; Fl 1–4.
G. samothracicus	Named in 2014; from the Aegean island of Samothrace in Greece; rare in the wild and in cultivation; similar to *G. nivalis*; Fl 1–2.
G. transcaucasicus	Named in 1909 by the Russian botanist Fomin from Azerbaijan; rare in the wild and in cultivation; broad green leaves similar to *G. woronowii;* Fl 12–4.
G. trojanus	Named in 2001 by Davis and Ozhatay from western Turkey; rare in the wild and in cultivation; similar to *G. nivalis* and *G. rizehensis*; Fl 1–3.
***G. woronowii (a)* or Woronow's snowdrop**	Named in 1935 by the Russian botanist Losina-Losinskaya, in honour of the plant collector Woronow; common in wild and cultivation; from Russia, Georgia and Turkey; bright green, wide leaves; Fl 1–4. (Figure 33).

CULTIVARS

Abington Green (s)	Discovered in the 1970s in Little Abington, Cambridgeshire by Blakeway-Phillips; bold green markings on the inner perianth segments (Figure 65).
Allenii (s)	A classic late snowdrop, noted for is strong scent – supposedly of bitter almonds (Figure 9); named by Baker in honour of James Allen in 1891; formerly thought to be a hybrid. DNA sequence evidence now suggests it is a variant of *G. alpinus;* has quite wide leaves, short and spreading at the time of flowering, with an attractive flower.
Anglesey Abbey (s)	An early, bright green, narrow-leaved snowdrop (Figure 23); as its name suggests, was found at Anglesey Abbey, a National Trust property near Lode, Cambridgeshire.

Anglesey Orange Tip (s)	An 'orange' tipped snowdrop, probably a cultivar of *G. elwesii,* with an orange glow at bud stage that can fade as the flowers open; a rare, fashionable and expensive snowdrop; from Anglesey Abbey, National Trust, Cambridgeshire in 2010.
Anne of Geierstein (s)	A late, quite rare, slow growing, desirable snowdrop, with thick outer perianth segments, named around 1900, probably by William Thomson after the novel of the same name by Walter Scott (Figure 10).
Atkinsii (s, a)	Named after Atkins, a Northampton nurseryman who, on retirement, moved to Painswick, Gloucestershire, where he received this classic, tall, early-flowering snowdrop, named after him by Allen in 1891. Often produces misshapen flowers, although the original stock was described as perfectly formed by Bowles in 1914.
Augustus (s, a)	Named after Bowles by Amy Doncaster before 1976 (Figure 32); a dwarf Crimean *G. plicatus*-type cultivar with heavily puckered flowers; leaves are characteristically oval in appearance, quite wide and with an obvious central white stripe, making this snowdrop easily recognizable; virus-free clones are available, although mine is probably potyvirus-infected because it occasionally shows yellowing and misshapen leaves.
Ballerina (d)	Found in Twigworth, Gloucestershire, by Phil Cornish in 1991 and listed by him in 2001; an attractive, short double giving the impression of a ballerina's tutu when in flower.
Barbara's Double (d)	Named in 1981 after the daughter, Lady Barbara Buchanan, of Lady Beatrix Stanley, who grew snowdrops in her garden at Sibbertoft Manor, Northamptonshire; said to have been collected by Bowles from Lady Beatrix Stanley's garden. A dainty, slow growing – but difficult snowdrop – with very regular doubling.
Benhall Beauty (s)	Raised by John Gray at Benhall, Suffolk, and named by Bowles in 1961; a tall, upright snowdrop, with distinctive inner perianth segment markings and a good scent (Figure 61).

Bertram Anderson (s, a)	Selected and named by Christopher Brickell from seedlings found in the late Anderson's garden in Lower Slaughter, Gloucestershire; an impressive large plant with well-developed outer perianth segments; available from 1992.
Bill Bishop (s)	A late-flowering snowdrop, found in Bill Bishop's garden in Herefordshire and named in 1998 by Christopher Brickell after him; a tall plant, it has enormous outer perianth segments; flowers may touch the ground.
Blewbury Tart (d)	An unusual freak double snowdrop found by Alan Street in the churchyard in the village of Blewbury, Oxfordshire; a very green-looking double with upward rather than the usual downward hanging flowers (Figure 52).
Blonde Inge (s)	An unusual 'half-yellow' snowdrop discovered in Germany by N. Top in a churchyard in Burscheid near Cologne in 1977; named after the old German song '*Wenn ich die Blonde Inge mit nach Hause bringe*' ('When I bring the blond Inge home with me'); a fairly small, common snowdrop-type cultivar that has a normal green ovary, but when the flower opens reveals yellow markings on the inner perianth segments (Figure 71), although in some flowers it is green.
Brenda Troyle (s)	A classic old favourite, recommended by Stern in 1956, of medium size not unlike 'S. Arnott' but differing in that the pedicel is longer than the spathe; origin of snowdrop and its name uncertain; scented (Figure 5 for inner perianth marks).
Cedric's Prolific (s)	Named after Cedric Morris – artist and plantsman – and found in his garden at Benton End House, Hadleigh, Suffolk; a strong-growing Elwes'-type snowdrop variant, with wide, glaucous green leaves and attractive, large flowers with good bold, inner perianth segment markings (Figure 66).
Cinderdine (s)	An Elwes'-type snowdrop found in 1996, with largish flowers (the outer perianth segments are likened to a small sailing boat) compared with the overall size of this plant; named after Daphne Chappell's cottage; she selected this snowdrop from H. Milford's garden at Chedworth, Gloucestershire.

Comet (s, a)	An Elwes'-type, tall, vigorous snowdrop named in 1986 by John Morley with long, arching pedicels and usually green stripes on the outer perianth segments near apex; leaves longer than 30 cm (Figure 44).
Cordelia (d)	A hybrid, raised and named by H. A. Greatorex of Blundall, Norwich, in the 1940s after a Shakespearean character in '*King Lear*'; usually a neat double (Figure 40). Bowles particularly admired this snowdrop; one of the later flowering Greatorex doubles.
Daglingworth (s)	A beautiful, late-flowering snowdrop with distinctive inner perianth markings, reminiscent of the slender, species snowdrop, *G. gracilis* (Figure 67); named after the village of Daglingworth in Gloucestershire where it was found by Ruth Birchall about 1990.
Daphne's Scissors (s)	Named after Daphne Chappell, who found this snowdrop in 1985 in Helen Milford's former garden in Chedworth, Gloucestershire, as a green-tipped *G. elwesii* variant. My clone, surprisingly, lacks these characteristic green tips but has the scissor-shaped green markings on the inner perianth segments.
David Shackleton (s)	A late, classic snowdrop, with distinct inner perianth segment markings; known since the 1960s; named after an Irish plantsman from Beech Park, Clonsilla, Co. Dublin (Figure 74); shows off its rather pointed flowers well clear of the shorter upright leaves.
Desdemona (d)	A hybrid, raised and named by H. A. Greatorex of Blundall, Norwich, in the 1940s; named after a Shakespearean character in '*Othello*'; often produces a third leaf from a single bulb, helping to distinguish it from the other Greatorex hybrids; Greatorex rated 'Desdemona' amongst the best of his doubles, alongside 'Ophelia'.
Diggory (s, a)	An immediately recognizable, must-have Crimean *G. plicatus*-type snowdrop, with distinctive ballooning and 'flat-bottomed', crinkled flowers (Figure 31); found by Rosie Steele and Richard Hobbs near Wells, Norfolk in 1993 and named after Diggory Birtles, Rosie's late son; its bulbs commanded very high prices when first introduced in 1998.

Dionysus (d)	A hybrid, raised and named by H. A. Greatorex of Blundall, Norwich, in the 1940s; named after the Greek god of wine and fertility; early flowering, tallish and said to produce occasional single and semi-double flowers, although I have not observed these aberrations myself.
Edith (s)	A quite rare, tall but slow to clump Elwes'-type snowdrop with Y-shaped markings on the inner perianth segments; named by Phil Cornish after his mother in 2001; not the easiest snowdrop.
Elfin (s)	A common snowdrop-type cultivar found by Phil Cornish in Wroxhall, Warwickshire, in 1997; a tiny snowdrop with green tips on the outer perianth segments.
Elizabeth Harrison (s)	A Woronow's-type snowdrop with a yellow ovary and yellow inner perianth segment markings introduced in 2012 by Ian Christie; a very fashionable and expensive yellow snowdrop; named after Elizabeth Harrison, in whose garden in Perthshire, Scotland it was found; said to be easy to grow.
Ex **Primrose Warburg 1** (d)	An unnamed, double snowdrop given to me by the late Primrose Warburg in about 1990; she did not identify it, hence my name; unlikely to be the same as the other doubles I grow in my garden.
Ex **Primrose Warburg 2** (d)	An unnamed, double snowdrop given me by the late Primrose Warburg in about 1990; she did not identify it, hence my name; differs from '*Ex* Primrose Warburg 1' in flowering later; unlikely to be the same as the other doubles I grow in my garden.
Faringdon Double (d)	An early-flowering 'semi-double'; flowers in December and is one of the first doubles to flower; found in the churchyard of Faringdon, Oxfordshire, in 1988 by Ruby and David Baker (Figures 21, 36).
Flore Pleno (d, a)	The common double snowdrop, also known as *G. nivalis* 'Flore Pleno'; first illustrated in the *Duchess of Beaufort's Flowers* by Kychicus,1703–1705 (Figures 15, 17).
Florence Baker (s)	Tall, early-flowering *G. plicatus* clone, very wide leaves (3.5 cm) and impressively large flowers; plants stand 25–30 cm tall; named by Ruth Stungo in Caroline and Michael Baker's garden, Gravesend, Kent; available from 1999.

G. Handel (s)	One of three Elwes'-type snowdrop, named after classical composers, with a light green leaf; flowers early in the New Year; selected by Leo Schoorl in 1986 from his garden at Lisse, The Netherlands, although originally from Turkey; said to bulk up well, but I find it is rather slow to produce offsets.
Galatea (s)	A classic, garden-worthy snowdrop originally named by James Allen in 1891, but modern stock may differ (Bishop, 2006), as it derives from uncertain stock from Ruth Birchall's garden in the 1970s; an excellent snowdrop with a long flower stalk, like 'Magnet', but differing in usually being kinked in the pedicel just behind the ovary (Figure 58).
Godfrey Owen (s, a)	A distinctive and very unusual snowdrop with six outer perianth and six inner perianth segments instead of the usual three; found and named in the mid-1990s by Margaret Owen near Wrentnall, Shrewsbury, Shropshire, and named after her husband.
Golden Fleece (s)	A yellow version of 'Trym' from Joe Sharman, the famous galanthophile; a hybrid of 'Trym' with 'Wendy's Gold' – a yellow Crimean *G. plicatus*-type snowdrop; a single bulb sold for £1,390 in 2015.
Green Necklace (s)	A common snowdrop *G. nivalis* cultivar found by Daphne Chappell in Ruth Birchall's garden, Cotswold Farm, Gloucestershire, in the 1970s; noted for its inner perianth segment markings reminiscent of a necklace.
Greenfields (s)	A late, reliable Irish snowdrop from the 1950s, of quite short stature; found by Liam Schofield in Greenfields – a neglected garden in Co. Tipperary, Ireland; inner perianth segments have broad, deep green marks.
Hiemalis (s, a)	A group of very early-flowering Elwes'-type snowdrops *G. elwesii,* mostly unnamed, but all are given the general name, 'Hiemalis', from the Latin meaning winter; very similar in appearance to the species snowdrop, *G. elwesii*, except they flower in late autumn (Figures 11, 20).
Highdown (s)	A cultivar of the slender snowdrop (*G. gracilis*) with narrow, somewhat twisted, grass-like leaves, a pale olive-green ovary and characteristic strong green

	markings on the inner perianth segments; named by Stern in about 1960 after his garden in Sussex.
Hill Poë (d)	A classic, late-flowering, diminutive, Irish snowdrop with near perfect doubling of the crowded inner perianth segments; described by James Hill Poë in his garden in Nenagh, Co. Tipperary, Ireland in about 1911; can be difficult to establish.
Hippolyta (d)	A hybrid, raised and named by H. A. Greatorex of Blundall, Norwich, in the 1940s, named after the mythological and Shakespearean character – the Queen of the Amazons – in '*A Midsummer Night's Dream*' (Figure 27); a very reliable, early, strong-growing double, although it does need splitting every 5–10 years; one of my favourite Greatorex doubles.
James Backhouse (s)	A variant of 'Atkinsii' with occasional aberrant flowers with four outer perianth segments and sometimes an odd-looking white bract just below the ovary; known for over 100 years; named after Backhouse of York; this clone and 'Atkinsii' in my garden also have occasional misshapen flowers, may have been muddled up in the past (Figure 14).
Jaquenetta (d)	A hybrid, raised and named by H. A. Greatorex of Blundall, Norwich, in the 1940s; named after the country woman in Shakespeare's '*Love's Labour's Lost*'; one of the most distinctive Greatorex hybrids; its outer petals are usually green-tipped which helps identification; very similar to 'Rodmarton', but distinguished by its thinner pedicel.
John Gray (s, a)	A classic, vigorous snowdrop with well-marked flowers; named in the 1960s by Anderson who collected this snowdrop from the garden of the late John Gray in Bentham, Suffolk; has large flowers on long pedicels so that flowers often droop down touching the soil (Figures 5, 56).
Ketton (s)	A classic, tall, strong snowdrop; introduced by Bowles in the 1950s from the village of Old Ketton, near Peterborough; unusually, has two pale green stains near the base of the inner perianth segments (Figures 5, 64).

Kite (s)	A desirable, strong-growing attractive snowdrop looking somewhat like a kite when fully open; occasionally produces aberrant double or twinned ovaries, with two flowers pressed against one another; selected by Oliver Wyatt as a seedling at Maidwell Hall, Northamptonshire, in the 1960s (Figures 5, 53, 54).
Lady Beatrix Stanley (d, a)	An early, classic double known since the 1950s, but named in 1981 by Richard Nutt after Lady Beatrix Stanley, who grew this snowdrop in her garden at Sibbertoft Manor, Northamptonshire; a rather squat snowdrop as it emerges, but then the flower stems unfold and shows off their double flowers with three very obvious, pointed outer petals; grows well in my lawn (Figures 24, 39).
Lady Elphinstone (d)	An unusual old yellow, double – very similar to 'Flore Pleno' – but with yellow markings instead of green, found by Sir Graham Elphinstone in Heawood Hall, Cheshire, in 1890; named by Samuel Arnott; said to be difficult to grow; has variable markings – green rather than yellow – in some years, but my clone is stable (Figure 70).
Lavinia (d)	A hybrid, raised and named by H. A. Greatorex of Blundall, Norwich, in the 1940s; distinctive because it is the latest of the Greatorex hybrids to flower in my garden; has a more dwarf habit than the other Greatorex hybrids I grow.
Little John (s)	A tall vigorous, upright cultivar with good inner perianth segment markings (Figure 5); originated from E. B. Anderson's garden in Lower Slaughter, Gloucestershire; named in the 1990s by Phil Cornish and Daphne Chappell.
Magnet (s, a)	A classic, must-have old cultivar known; named by James Allen in 1888; its arched flowers are held on the end of a long and slender pedicel that nods in the wind (Figures 5, 26).
Maidwell L (s)	A vigorous widely grown Elwes'-type cultivar that flowers early; selected and named by Oliver Wyatt at Maidwell Hall School, Northamptonshire (Figure 43).

Mandarin (s)	A robust snowdrop with an olive-green ovary; found in a garden in Longlevens, Gloucestershire, by Phil Cornish in the 1990s and named for its oriental-like appearance (Figure 72).
Margaret Biddulph (s)	Has prominent green markings on its outer perianth segments; named by Simon Biddulph, Rodmarton Manor, Gloucestershire for his grandmother (Figure 12).
Mary Biddulph (s)	A strong-growing Elwes'-type cultivar; named by Daphne Chappell around 2000 after Mary Biddulph, who was a galanthophile, gardening at Rodmarton Manor, Gloucestershire, in the 1960–1970s; originally selected by Oliver Wyatt (Figure 42).
Merlin (s, a)	A classic old-fashioned variety named by James Allen in 1891 and noted for its nearly completely green inner perianth segments; slow to bulk up compared to many modern varieties (Figure 5).
Mighty Atom (s)	An old favourite with very large flowers; a so-called dumpy snowdrop, flowering close to the soil; named in the 1960s by E. B. Anderson and Fred Buglass, who collected this snowdrop from the garden of the late John Gray in Bentham, Suffolk (Figure 68).
Miller's Late (s)	A classic late-flowering snowdrop as the name suggests; a rather short plant at the time of flowering; has wide leaves and a well-developed arching spathe; available from 1967; unknown who the Miller was (Figure 75).
Modern Art (s)	A strong, very upright, green-tipped snowdrop introduced around 1960, probably by E. B. Anderson (Figure 62).
Mrs McNamara (s, a)	An outstanding, early and tall Elwes'-type cultivar with large, impressive flowers; named in 1996 by Christopher Brickell after Dylan Thomas' mother-in-law (Figure 22).
Mrs Thompson (s)	The best known of all the aberrant snowdrops, producing all sorts of distinctly odd features (Figure 55), such as variable number of outer petals (up to 6), ovary doubling and even normal-looking flowers; Mrs Thompson, from Escrick, York, found this freakish plant around 1950.

Natalie Garton (d)	A semi-double with the broad, glaucous green leaves typical of an Elwes'-type cultivar; named after Natalie Garton of Ramsden, Oxfordshire, around 1995.
Nerissa (d)	A hybrid, raised and named by H. A. Greatorex of Blundall, Norwich, in the 1940s; the name of Portia's lady-in-waiting in Shakespeare's '*The Merchant of Venice*'. Bowles, writing in Stern's *Snowdrops and Snowflakes* (1956), particularly admired 'Nerissa'.
Ophelia (d)	One of the best known, early-flowering hybrids named by H. A. Greatorex of Blundall, Norwich, in the 1940s; 'Ophelia' was one of his best hybrids – along with 'Desdemona', according to Greatorex; named after the character in Shakespeare's '*Hamlet*'.
Peg Sharples (s)	A classic snowdrop widely grown for its late-flowering habit and attractive flowers with good markings; named by Richard Nutt, who stated it was raised by Peg Sharples, Grange-over-Sands, Cumbria in the 1960s from seed supplied by E. B. Anderson.
Primrose Warburg (s)	A famous yellow snowdrop; collected by fellow galanthophiles from the late Primrose Warburg's South Hayes, Oxfordshire garden and named after her in 1997; possibly virus-infected (Figure 69).
Pusey Green Tips (d)	A rather diminutive 'Flore Pleno'-type double with distorted inner florets, selected because of the obvious green tips on the outer florets; probably originated from the village of Pusey, Oxfordshire in 1938.
Richard Ayres (d)	An early-flowering double, named by the National Trust after the former head gardener at their garden at Anglesey Abbey, Cambridgeshire in 1987; distinctive in having four, and sometimes more, rather obvious projecting, outer flower segments.
Robin Hood (s)	A long-established cultivar, very upright-looking and strong-growing which bulks up well; named originally by James Allen in 1891 but modern stock from Bowles probably different (Figure 45).
Rodmarton (d)	A very green double, only subtly different from the Greatorex hybrid 'Jaquenetta'; found and named by Mary Biddulph at Rodmarton Manor, Gloucestershire, in the mid-1970s.

Rodmarton Capella (s)	A tall Rodmarton snowdrop with broad leaves and very dark green inner flower markings, although not as tall as 'Rodmarton Regulus'; selected by Simon Biddulph of Rodmarton Manor, Gloucestershire, around 2000 (Figure 49).
Rodmarton Regulus (s)	A magnificent, very tall, early Elwes'-type cultivar; the tallest snowdrop cultivar I know of, with exceedingly large flowers, and very long, impressive leaves after flowering; selected by Simon Biddulph of Rodmarton Manor, Gloucestershire, around 2000 (Figure 25).
Rodmarton Sirius (s)	A medium height snowdrop with very distinctive inner flower markings and an olive-green ovary characteristic of the slender snowdrop *G. gracilis;* selected by Simon Biddulph of Rodmarton Manor, Gloucestershire, around 2000 (Figure 48).
S. Arnott (s, a)	A classic, strongly scented, must-have cultivar known for over a century; named in 1951 after Samuel Arnott, who likely raised this cultivar and sent it to Henry John Elwes of Colesbourne, Gloucestershire, around 1920; initially distributed as 'Arnott's seedling' (Figures 5, 29).
Sally Ann (s)	Has good inner flower markings with a thick green cross; found by Herbert Ransom and E. B. Anderson in Mathias' garden, Hyde Lodge, Chalford Gloucestershire; named in the late 1950s after one of Herbert Ransom's daughters (Figure 73).
Sandersii (s)	A diminutive, but charming common snowdrop variant with a yellow ovary and yellow markings on the inner perianth segments; named by H. Harpur-Crewe as *G. nivalis* var. *sandersii* after Mr Sanders of Newnham, Cambridge, who found it in Northumberland around 1876; the first of the yellows to be named (Figure 59).
Scharlockii (s)	A classic, quirky cultivar with a spathe (the original membranous covering of the flower) that splits into two separate long and curved green leaf-like structures, giving it an unusual appearance resembling miniature, elongated donkey's ears; has green-tipped outer flower segments; named in 1868 after the pharmacist, Jules Scharlock who found it in Germany.

Sibbertoft Manor (s)	A very attractive, large and sturdy snowdrop; named in 1999 by Ronald Mackenzie, who found it in the famous Sibbertoft Bank in the garden of the late snowdrop enthusiast, Primrose Warburg, in Oxfordshire (Figure 47).
South Hayes (s, a)	A much sought-after, unusual cultivar named in honour of the late Primrose Warburg's Oxfordshire garden, where it was discovered in the early 1990s, probably as a seedling of 'Trym'; like 'Trym', it has abnormal flowers with the outer perianth segments replaced by a whorl in appearance not unlike the inner perianth segments; 'South Hayes' has an 'exclamation-like' green mark on its outer flower segment that differs from 'Trym' and 'Trimmer', which boast only a single mark.
Spindlestone Surprise (s, a)	One of the best yellow snowdrops; similar to 'Primrose Warburg'; originated in Diana Aitchison's garden at Spindlestone, Belford, Northumberland; named in 1998 (Figure 30).
St Anne's (s)	An attractive, late, very upright snowdrop, with pointed rather than rounded outer flower segments and good inner markings; found in Norfolk; known since 1989 and named after St Anne's Manor, Sutton Bonnington, Nottinghamshire, once the home of Lady Barbara Buchanan, the daughter of Lady Beatrix Stanley (Figure 76).
Straffan (s, a)	A classic Crimean *G. plicatus*-type cultivar, with largish, rounded flowers; selected because it commonly produces two scapes (flower stalks) from one bulb; the third-oldest snowdrop variety still grown; originally from Straffan House, Co. Kildare, Ireland, although date of origin uncertain, either 1858 or around 1875 (Figures 5, 57).
Three leaves (s, a)	An early, attractive, strong-growing Elwes'-type cultivar with three leaves instead of the usual two; as the outer perianth segments mature, they become distinctly long and pointed; known since 1993.
Titania (d)	A late-flowering hybrid, raised and named by H. A. Greatorex of Blundall, Norwich, in the 1940s; the name of a character in Shakespeare's '*A Midsummer Night's Dream*'.

Trimmer (s)	An earlier flowering seedling of Trym; selected by Rob and Rannveig Wallis from their garden in Carmarthenshire, Wales around 2010; an unusual, but very desirable snowdrop with shorter outer petals marked with two separate green marks (Figure 60).
Trym (s)	A famous, must-have snowdrop originating in the garden of Jane Gibbs; named after the village Westbury on Trym near Bristol where it was found in the 1980s; name suggested by Christopher Brickell; unusually, the outer flower petals are short and boldly marked in green, closely resembling the inner ones. When mature the outer segments of the flower curl out resembling the eaves of a Chinese pagoda.
Tubby Merlin (s)	Named in the 1960s by E. B. Anderson of Lower Slaughter Gloucestershire; like 'Merlin', this has an almost complete green inner marking on the inner perianth segments; still regarded as a good snowdrop, clumping up well.
Warei (s)	Originally thought to be a seedling of 'Scharlockii' because of its long, elongated spathe, it is quite small with green-tipped flowers and a very long pedicel that droops in a characteristic way; named after Thomas Ware of Tottenham, London in 1886 (Figure 63).
Warham (s)	A classic snowdrop; found in a garden in Warham, Norfolk by Rev. C. Digby; sent to Bowles in 1916; possibly originally introduced from Crimea about 1855; vigorous, with broad leaves and a stripe on the upper surface – not unlike 'Augustus' – but with more upright leaves.
Washfield Colesbourne (s)	An elegant snowdrop with strong green markings covering most of the inner petals; named after Elizabeth Strangman's Washfield Nursery, Hawkhurst, Kent, as a seedling of 'Colesbourne' around 1980; slow to multiply.
Wasp (s)	A very fine snowdrop, discovered in 1995 by Veronica Cross in the former Backhouse Garden at Sutton Court, Herefordshire; quite delicate-looking cultivar that clumps up well, with slender leaves and a very pointed flower that resembles a wasp in flight (Figures 5, 37, 38).

Wendy's Gold (s)	A strong Crimean-type cultivar with a yellow ovary and yellow markings on the inner perianth segments; found at Wandlebury Ring, Cambridgeshire by the Warden, Bill Clark, in 1974 and named later after his wife; possibly virus-infected (Figures 5, 50).
White Swan (d)	One of the less well-known, but elegant hybrids raised and named by H. A. Greatorex of Blundall, Norwich, in the 1940s; praised by Bowles in 1956 as one of the best Greatorex hybrids (Figures 28, 46).
Winifrede Mathias (s)	An old-fashioned, medium-sized cultivar; found in Hyde Lodge, Chalford, Gloucestershire, by Herbert Ransom and E. B. Anderson in the late 1950s; named after the snowdrop enthusiast, Mrs Mathias.
Yvonne Hay (s)	An Elwes'-type cultivar with wide, glaucous green leaves and attractive, large flowers with good bold, inner markings; named around 1999 by Harry Hay of Margery Hall Farm, Surrey, after his wife.

EIGHT

FAMOUS GALANTHOPHILES

Interest in growing snowdrops is not a new phenomenon. Indeed the word 'galanthophile', now widely used, is reputed to have been used by Bowles writing to Wyatt in 1956.[104]

Victorian gardeners were fascinated by snowdrops and collected and named different species and varieties. Here I record a few of the more famous snowdrop enthusiasts of the past, many of whom have snowdrops named after them.[105]

Allen, James (1832–1906)

Allen was an early galanthophile who, in 1891, read a paper at the RHS Snowdrop Conference, noting over 100 different snowdrop seedlings in his Somerset garden. Famously, the almond-scented snowdrop, 'Allenii', was named after him. Often referred to as *Galanthus* X *allenii* – indicating a hybrid – DNA sequencing[106] now suggests it is a variety of the alpine snowdrop, *G. alpinus*.

Arnott, Samuel (1852–1930)

Arnott was a writer and gardener. The strongly fragrant snowdrop 'S. Arnott' was named after him in 1951. Originally sent by Arnott to Henry John Elwes at Colesbourne, it was further redistributed as 'Arnott's seedling'.

Atkins, James (1804–1884)

Atkins was a Northampton nurseryman who, on retirement, moved to Painswick, Gloucestershire, where he received the tall, early-flowering snowdrop, 'Atkinsii', named after him in 1891.

Baker, John Gilbert (1834–1920)

Baker was an eminent Kew botanist, who named several snowdrops including 'Allenii' after James Allen, and *G. plicatus* ssp. *byzantinus*.

Biddulph, Mary (1909–1991)

Biddulph established a snowdrop garden at Rodmarton Manor, Gloucestershire, in a formal setting of stonework and terrace adjacent to the Manor in the 1960s and 1970s. She found the snowdrop 'Rodmarton', and 'Mary Biddulph' is named after her. Her son, Simon Biddulph, has extended the collection and introduced other fine snowdrops from Rodmarton, including 'Margaret Biddulph' and 'Rodmarton Regulus'.

Bowles, Edward Augustus (1865–1954)

Bowles was an authority on and painter of snowdrops, who wrote a chapter in Stern's book *Snowdrops and Snowflakes* published in 1956. In that book he described the snowdrops he liked best. He corresponded with other snowdrop enthusiasts over a period of about 70 years. 'Augustus' is named after him.

Elwes, Henry John (1846–1922)

Elwes, an explorer and plant hunter, introduced the snowdrop *G. elwesii* (named after him by Hooker in 1875) from Turkey to his garden in Colesbourne, Gloucestershire. His great grandson, Sir Henry Elwes and Lady Caroline, have extended the collection of snowdrops in Colesbourne. This garden has one of most extensive snowdrop collections open to the public in the UK.

Greatorex, Heyrick (1884–1954)

Greatorex was an unconventional man, who hybridized the *G. nivalis* 'Flore Pleno' double snowdrop with the more vigorous Crimean snowdrop *G. plicatus,* to create 12 or more vigorous doubles, which he named mostly after Shakespearean characters.

Ransom, Herbert (1909–1985)

Gardener for Leonard and Winifrede Mathias of the Giant Snowdrop Company, he and Edward Anderson named the snowdrops 'Sally Ann' after his daughter, 'Armine' after the Mathias' daughter and 'Winifrede Mathias' after his employer. All three snowdrops are still available.

Stanley, Beatrix (1877–1944)

Lady Beatrix Stanley grew snowdrops at her garden at Sibbertoft Manor, Northamptonshire. The early, distinctive double 'Lady Beatrix Stanley' is named after her, while the more dainty, double 'Barbara's Double' is named after her daughter. After Lady Beatrix's death, Primrose Warburg collected snowdrops from Sibbertoft Manor in Northamptonshire and planted them on Sibbertoft Bank in her own Oxfordshire garden. The snowdrop 'Sibbertoft Manor' was named after Lady Beatrix Stanley's Northamptonshire garden.

Stern, Frederick (1884–1967)

Stern is best known as the author of the first snowdrop 'bible' – *Snowdrops and snowflakes* published in 1956. Although now out of date, it is a useful historical survey of snowdrops grown in the UK, some now sadly lost. He grew a number of snowdrops in his garden in Highdown, Sussex, e.g. *G. gracilis* 'Highdown'.

Warburg, Primrose (1920–1996)

Primrose Warburg was an enthusiastic collector of snowdrops in her South Hayes garden near Oxford. Famously, she did not always label (or she lost the labels) of snowdrops that she collected. When I bought two different 'doubles' from her on an open day in the early 1990s, I resorted to naming them: '*ex* Primrose Warburg 1' and '*ex* Primrose Warburg 2'. I have still not identified these 'doubles'. After her death, Ronald Mackenzie found a new, yellow snowdrop in her garden, which was named 'Primrose Warburg' after her. 'South Hayes' is another famous snowdrop found there and named after Primrose Warburg's garden.

Wyatt, Oliver (1898–1973)

Wyatt created a garden at Maidwell Hall School, Northamptonshire, where he was headmaster. 'Maidwell L', amongst others, was selected from this garden. He also named 'Kite', which was found as a seedling there.

Appendix 1: Buying snowdrops

The common snowdrop (*G. nivalis*), its double form 'Flore Pleno', Elwes' snowdrop (*G. elwesii*) and Woronow's snowdrop (*G. woronowii*) are now generally available from many garden suppliers as pot grown plants from January onwards. (Or from June in Australia and New Zealand).

Below is a selection of specialist snowdrop suppliers in the UK, Ireland, The Netherlands, Germany, Belgium, Canada, USA, Australia and New Zealand. If visiting in person, check the website as opening times may be restricted. Some nurseries supply by mail order only and some only supply bulbs.

Note that snowdrops (*Galanthus*) can be confused with snowflakes (*Leucojum*).

UK

- ***Ashwood Nurseries****, West Midlands, DY6 0AE www.ashwoodnurseries.com*
- ***Avon Bulbs****, Somerset, TA13 5HE www.avonbulbs.co.uk*
- ***Beth Chatto Gardens****, Essex, CO7 7DB www.bethchatto.co.uk*
- ***Bloms Bulbs****, Bedfordshire, MX44 1ZZ, bulbs only www.blomsbulbs.com*
- ***Broadleigh Gardens****, Somerset, TA4 1AE www.broadleighbulbs.co.uk*
- ***Cambo Estate****, Fife, KY16 8QD cambosnowdrops.com*
- ***Colesbourne Park****, Gloucestershire, GL53 9NP www.colesbournegardens.org.uk*
- ***Edrom Nurseries****, Berwickshire, TD14 5TZ www.edrom-nurseries.co.uk*
- ***Elworthy Cottage****, Somerset, TA4 3PX www.elworthy-cottage.co.uk*
- ***Evenley Wood Garden****, Northamptonshire, NN13 5SH No mail order www.evenleywoodgarden.co.uk*
- ***Foxgrove Plants****, Berkshire, RG14 6RE www.foxgroveplants.co.uk*
- ***Harveys garden Plants****, Suffolk, IP31 3SJ www.harveysgardenplants.co.uk*
- ***Monksilver Nursery****, Cambridgeshire, CB24 8TW www.monksilvernursery.co.uk*

- ***North Green Snowdrops**, Suffolk, NR34 8DG www.northgreensnowdrops.co.uk.*
- ***P. de Jager**, Kent, ME17 1DW, bulbs only www.dejager.co.uk*
- ***Pottertons Nursery**, Lincolnshire, LN7 6HX www.pottertons.co.uk*
- ***Rare Plants**, Wrexham, Clwyd, bulbs only www.rareplants.co.uk*
- ***Rodmarton Manor**, Gloucestershire, GL7 6PF, www.rodmarton-manor.co.uk, Email: enquiries@rodmarton-manor.co.uk.*
- ***Sarah Raven's Kitchen Garden**, Wiltshire, SN8 4AN, www.sarahraven.com*
- ***Snape Cottage**, Dorset, SP8 5BZ, www.snapecottage.co.uk*
- ***Thompson & Morgan**, Ipswich, IP8 3BU www.thompson-morgan.com*

Ireland

- ***Field of Blooms**, Nenagh, Co. Tipperary, Ireland, www.fieldofblooms.ie*
- ***Timpany Nurseries**, Co. Down, BT24 8PA, Northern Ireland, www.timpanynurseries.com*

The Netherlands

- ***Bloms Bulbs**, limited snowdrop bulb stock online, www.bulbi.nl*
- ***De Boschhoeve Garden**, Wolfheze, snowdrop festival in February to view and buy, good selection, www.boschhoeve.nl*

Germany

- ***Garten in den Wiesen**, Cottbus, Brandenburg, good selection of snowdrops www.engelmanii.de*
- ***Botanical garden in Nettetal**, North-Rhine Westphalia, extensive snowdrop collection, www.oirlicherblumengarten.de*

Belgium

- ***Koen van Poucke**, Sint-Niklaas, good selection, www.koenvanpoucke.be*
- ***Alpine Plants Cathy Porter**, Bruges, www.alpenplanten.be*
- ***National Botanic Garden of Belgium**, Meisse, www.br.fgov.be*

USA

- ***Holland Bulb Farms**, Milwaukee, WI, limited Dutch imported snowdrop bulbs, www.hollandbulbfarms.com*
- ***Van Engelen/John Scheepers**, Bantam, CT, limited Dutch imported snowdrop bulbs, www.johnscheepers.com*
- ***Edgwood**, Exton, PA, extensive specialist collection of potted dormant snowdrop cultivars and species, online orders only, www.edgwoodgardens.net*

- ***Carolyn's Shade Gardens***, *Bryn Mawr, PA, extensive specialist selection for pick up or mail order, www.carolynshadegardens.com*

Canada

- ***Campbell River Garden Centre***, *Campbell, BC, bulbs, www.crgardencentre.com*

Australia

- ***Clover Hill Rare Plants***, *Katoomba, NSW, extensive collection of specialist snowdrops, www.cloverhillrareplants.com.au*

New Zealand

- ***Blue Mountain Nurseries***, *Tapanui, a reasonable collection of snowdrops, www.bmn.co.nz*
- ***Maple Glen Plants***, *Wyndham, variety of potted snowdrops, www.mapleglen.co.nz*
- ***Hokonui Alpines***, *Southland, a couple of potted snowdrops, mail order, www.hokonuialpines.co.nz*

Appendix 2: Looking at Snowdrops

Galanthophiles like to admire snowdrop collections in other people's gardens. Many owners and organizations now open their gardens in February for snowdrop enthusiasts to visit. These may be big estates, such as properties owned by the National Trust or other charities, but now also include smaller gardens open under the National Garden Scheme (yellow book). These are definitely worth visiting. Often a few choice snowdrops will be available to buy.

Below are just a few of the many gardens to visit in the UK and Ireland. Check websites online for opening times.

- *Altamont Garden, Co. Carlow, Ireland*
- *Anglesey Abbey, Cambridgeshire (National Trust)*
- *Brandy Mount House, New Alresford, Hampshire (National Garden Scheme)*
- *Cambo Estates, Fife*
- *Castle Kennedy Gardens, Dumfries and Galloway*
- *Chelsea Physic Garden, London*
- *Colesbourne Park, Gloucestershire*
- *Cotswold Farm Garden, Gloucestershire*
- *Dawyck Botanic Gardens, Peebles, Scottish Borders*
- *Dunvegan Castle and Gardens, Skye*
- *Evenley Wood Garden, Northamptonshire*
- *Fyvie Castle, Aberdeenshire*
- *Logan Botanic Garden, Dumfries*
- *Painswick Rococo Gardens, Gloucestershire*
- *Rodmarton Manor, Gloucestershire*
- *Royal Botanic Gardens, Kew, London*
- *Royal Botanic Gardens, Edinburgh*

- *Royal Horticultural Society Gardens, Surrey*
- *Scone Palace, Perthshire*
- *Waterperry Gardens, Oxfordshire*
- *Welford Park, Berkshire*

Appendix 3: Tables listing double and single snowdrops

There may be as many as 2,000 different snowdrop cultivars, and 22 species, now described, such is the popularity of snowdrop collectors and the enthusiasm of snowdrop collectors and breeders to bring new cultivars onto the market.

The list of snowdrops in Table 3 (doubles) and Table 4 (singles) list those species or cultivars mentioned in this book for the convenience of readers.

Table 3 Double snowdrops

Ballerina	Jaquenetta
Barbara's Double	Lady Beatrix Stanley
Blewbury Tart	Lady Elphinstone
Cordelia	Lavinia
Desdemona	Natalie Garton
Dionysus	Nerissa
Ex Primrose Warburg 1	Ophelia
Ex Primrose Warburg 2	Pusey Green Tips
Faringdon Double	Richard Ayres
Flore Pleno	Rodmarton
Hill Poë	Titania
Hippolyta	White Swan

Table 4 Single snowdrops

Abington Green	*G. krasnovii*	Mary Biddulph
Allenii	*G. lagodechianus*	Merlin
Anglesey Abbey	*G. nivalis*	Mighty Atom
Anglesey Orange Tip	*G. panjutinii*	Miller's Late
Anne of Geierstein	*G. peshmenii*	Modern Art
Atkinsii	*G. platyphyllus*	Mrs McNamara
Augustus	*G. plicatus*	Mrs Thompson
Benhall Beauty	*G. plicatus 'plicatus'*	Peg Sharples
Bertram Anderson	*G. reginae-olgae*	Primrose Warburg
Bill Bishop	*G. reginae-olgae 'Cambridge'*	Robin Hood
Blonde Inge	*G. reginae-olgae 'vernalis'*	Rodmarton Capella
Brenda Troyle	*G. rizehensis*	Rodmarton Regulus
Cedric's Prolific	*G. samothracicus*	Rodmarton Sirius
Cinderdine	*G. transcaucasicus*	S. Arnott
Comet	*G. trojanus*	Sally Ann
Daglingworth	*G. woronowii*	Sandersii
Daphne's Scissors	G. Handel	Scharlockii
David Shackleton	Galatea	Sibbertoft Manor
Diggory	Godfrey Owen	South Hayes
Edith	Golden Fleece	Spindlestone Surprise
Elfin	Green Necklace	St Anne's
Elizabeth Harrison	Greenfields	Straffan
Florence Baker	Hiemalis	Three Leaves
G. alpinus	Highdown	Trimmer
G. alpinus 'bortkewitsch-ianus'	James Backhouse	Trym
G. angustifolius	John Gray	Tubby Merlin
G. bursanus	Ketton	Warei
G. cilicicus	Kite	Warham
G. elwesii	Little John	Washfield Colesbourne
G. fosteri	Magnet	Wasp
G. gracilis	Maidwell L	Wendy's Gold
G. ikariae	Mandarin	Winifrede Mathias
G. koenenianus	Margaret Biddulph	Yvonne Hay

Endnotes

Foreword

1 *The Burning of the Leaves*, Laurence Binyon (1869–1943), poet.

Preface

2 'Of Bulbous Violets' from Gerard, J. (1633), pp. 147 and 149.

3 *See* Davis, A. P. (1999); Bishop, M., Davis, A., Grimshaw J. (2006); Cox, F. (2018); Slade, N. (2014).

Chapter One

4 *See* Stern, F. C. (1956), p. 65.

5 *See* Davis, A. P. (1999), p. 86. The main evidence that the snowdrop is not native to Britain is that the range of variation seen in British *G. nivalis* is less than that seen in indigenous populations in central and eastern Europe.

6 *See* Gerard, J. (1633), p. 147, left woodcut, labelled 'Timely flouring bulbous Violet'. Gerard does not retain the Latin name previously used by Dodoens (1568) (see note 8), although the woodcut is identical.

7 *See* Gunther R. T. (1922), p. 311, where 'Snowe Dropps' are listed as growing in 1615 in the garden of Richard Shanne of Yorkshire.

8 Dodoens', L'Obel's and L'Ecluse's herbals were all published by Plantin in Antwerp; the same snowdrop woodcut, retained by the publisher, was reused. Gerard's herbal of 1597 reproduces a different snowdrop woodcut (borrowed from the Frankfurt publishers of Tabernaemontanus's *Eicones Plantarum*, 1590), although the later, much enlarged, Johnson's second edition of Gerard's herbal in 1633 uses the earlier Plantin image of the snowdrop. Most of Johnson's woodcuts, published in London, made use of the Plantin woodcuts. Indeed, Johnson in his preface, admits this. He states: 'Now I come to particulars, and first of figures: I have, as I said, made use of those wherewith the Workes of Dodonaeus, Lobel and Clusius were formerly printed…' Thus the woodcuts of the common snowdrop (*G. nivalis*) in Figure 2 (from Gerard, 1633) and Figure 77 (from Dodoens, 1568) – are the same, but the caption naming the snowdrop (in Latin) differs. However, a similar Latin caption is in use in Figure 3 (from Gerard,1633) and Figure 79 (from L'Ecluse, 1601) for identical woodcuts of the Crimean snowdrop (*G. plicatus*). A letter dated 26 August 1632 (*see* Imhof, D., 2001, pp. 179–190) from Balthasar Moretus to Richard Whitaker, publisher of Gerard (1633), makes it clear that the woodcuts were shipped from

Antwerp to London. The letter states 'Je vous ay envoyé a vos correspondents a Duynkercke Guillaume Randale and Jean Ardin une balle de la marque en marge (No. 5RW), en laquelle sont mises 21 boites pleines des figures de Dodonaeus, avec celles de Lobel & Clusius qui sont adioustees au Dodonaeus en flamen: & ce suivant l'ordre & accord faict le Sr. Leonel Wack, lequel m'a promis de payer ceste sepmaine 600 florin pour l'usage d'icelles au votre Herbier Anglois.' Freely translated as, '*I have arranged to send you, via agents William Randale and Jean Ardin in Dunkirk, a bale of 21 full boxes of Dodonaeus' woodblocks together with those of Lobel and Clusius which are contained with those of Dodonaeus in Flemish. Following this order, the merchant Leonel Wack has promised to pay me this week 600 florins for their use in your English Herbal.*' A total of 2,997 woodblocks were shipped, according to Imhof. Note that Leonel Wack was acting as a financial intermediary between Moretus and Whitaker. In subsequent letters, Moretus repeatedly asked, without success, for his woodblocks to be returned promptly, as he needed them for a Dutch herbal of Dodonaeus in preparation. But he had to wait 4 years before they were returned in 1636. Even then, it was later discovered in 1642, that three woodblocks were missing. Whitaker then admitted he had lost these woodblocks, requiring Balthasar II Moretus (Balthasar Moretus had died by then) to have them recut.

9 *See* Pratt, A. (1873) p. 239 of vol. V. Pratt suggested monks probably introduced the snowdrop into Britain. She adds that the snowdrop was 'deemed…an emblem of feminine purity – one of its old names being "Fair Maid of February"'.

10 Parkinson, J. (1629), p. 109. The legend to the multifigured plate on p. 107 lists *Leucojum bulbosum praecox minus* (now *G. nivalis)* but does not illustrate it.

11 L'Ecluse, C. (Clusius) (1601).

12 Dodoens R. (1586). The term 'violet' did not necessarily refer to a violet-coloured flower. It was a general term; there was no inconsistency in calling a plant a 'white violet'. Indeed, Pliny in the first century AD, refers to some violets as 'Viola alba'. These may well have been the snowflake, *Leucojum vernum*.

13 Blunt, W. (1950) pp. 8–9.

14 Sowerby, J. (1790–1814).

15 Snowdrops *(Galanthus)* are distinguished from snowflakes (*Leucojum)* by having six unequal flower, or perianth segments; the inner segments are half the length of the outer segments. In snowflakes, the six flower segments are of equal length.

16 Davis, A. P. (1999). *See* pp. 77–79 for details.

17 Davis, A. P. (1999). *See* pp. 77–79 for details.

18 Zubov, D. A., Konka, Y., Davis, A. P. (2019).

19 Ronsted, N., Zubov, D., Bruun-Lund, S., Davis, A. P. (2013). DNA sequence data for a part of the ribosomal DNA was used in this report. This analysis did not include *G. samothracicus* and *G. bursanus*, described only later in 2014 and 2019, respectively.

20 Examples of subspecies occur in the Crimean snowdrop (*G. plicatus),* which has been split into two subspecies, *plicatus* and *byzantinus.* These two subspecies differ only in one quite subtle, but distinctive feature: the extent of the green marking on the inner perianth segment. There is a single green mark in subspecies *plicatus* but two green marks in subspecies *byzantinus.* Another example, where subspecies

have been recognized is in the autumn flowering snowdrop, Queen Olga's snowdrop (*G. reginae-olgae*). This snowdrop occurs as subspecies *reginae-olgae*, which is the earlier flowering subspecies with no leaves visible at flowering, or subspecies *vernalis*, which flowers later with visible leaves.

21 Davis, A. P. (1999). See pp. 77–79 for details.

22 Davis, A. P. (1999). See pp. 77–79 for details.

23 Recognizing this, some snowdrop suppliers, e.g. Colesbourne Park, Gloucestershire, have used the name, *G. hybridus*, followed by the name of the variety or cultivar.

24 Stern, F. C. (1956) pp. 69–70 in an included article by E. A. Bowles.

25 My naming approach is similar to Cox, F. (2018) in her snowdrop index, except I omit the symbol '*G*'.

Chapter Two

26 On planting a batch of 24 dried bulbs from a well-known supplier of the common snowdrop (*G. nivalis*) in pots in mid-November, I found that only 18 bulbs produced flowers or a visible foliage by mid-February. Even then, two bulbs turned out, unexpectedly, to be the double form of the common snowdrop *G. nivalis* 'Flore Pleno', illustrating the risk of growing an incorrect snowdrop bulb.

27 As explained in Chapter One, I have simplified the naming of snowdrops by abbreviating the genus (*Galanthus*, abbreviated *G.*) and in many cases the species because this is often merely conjecture rather than proven. Many cultivars are naturally occurring seedlings or hybrids where the parental species are not known with certainty. In this case, *Galanthus X allenii* was formerly regarded as a probable hybrid, but recent DNA sequencing suggests it is simply a cultivar of the species *G. alpinus* (*see* Chapter One). In agreement with its stated origin from the Caucasus by Baker, who originally named it in 1891, I have omitted the symbol '*X*' implying a hybrid and simply used the cultivar name 'Allenii'.

28 'Anne of Geierstein' is my abbreviation of *Galanthus* 'Anne of Geierstein'.

29 *See* Bishop, M., Davis, A. P., Grimshaw, J. (2006), pp. 314–317 for a description of twin-scaling.

30 Stern, F. C. (1956), p. 78.

31 *See* Bishop, M., Davis, A. P., Grimshaw, J. (2006), pp. 311–312.

32 Stern, F. C. (1956), p. 78.

33 *See* Bishop, M., Davis, A. P., Grimshaw, J. (2006), pp. 325–327. Leaf scorch (*Stagonospora curtisii*, recently renamed *Peyronellaea curtisii)* may be the most serious disease of snowdrops. It is well known in daffodils and other species within the *Amaryllidaceae*, where it is known as leaf scorch or tip burn. The fungus first attacks the flowers and leaves, but this may not be visible initially. Only in the second year is a brownish scorch mark present at the tip or on the sides of the leaves. Further rounds of infection cause the fungal spores to attack the base of the leaves, transferring the infection to the bulb, which can then quickly kill the plant. Another fungus, *Botrytis galanthina*, is specific to snowdrops. Other fungi, *Sclerotinia gladioli*, or 'fire' of gladioli, and *Botryotinia narcissicola*, or 'smoulder', cause severe stunting and yellowing of foliage, and the mycelium eventually infects the bulb which becomes soft.

34 *See* Bishop, M., Davis, A. P., Grimshaw J. (2006), p. 323. Insect pests can kill snowdrops. They include the larvae of the common swift moth (*Hepialus lupulinus*) and the large *Merodon equestris*, and also small narcissus flies, *Eumerus strigatus* and *Eumerus tuberculatus*.

35 *See* Bishop, M., Davis, A. P., Grimshaw J. (2006) p. 325. Potato Y virus is of commercial importance because it infects potatoes and other crops. It is a well-characterized, relatively simple RNA (ribonucleic acid)-containing virus.

36 To investigate whether viruses are widespread in snowdrops, it is not necessary to isolate new viruses *per se* from potentially infected plants. It would be easier to use modern DNA sequencing methods to search for the genome of a suspected virus first. In a research environment, it is not difficult to isolate DNA or RNA from snowdrop leaves or bulbs by using commercially available kits. After copying the RNA sequences into DNA with enzymes, the resultant DNA could then be sequenced in a dedicated sequencing facility for large-scale genomic DNA sequencing. Though costly at the moment (about £2,000), analysis of the resultant DNA sequence information, which requires specialist bioinformatic skills, would then establish whether there are sequences similar to known, previously sequenced RNA plant viruses, such as Potato Y virus or other known plant viruses. Of course snowdrop-specific viruses would not be discovered by this whole genome sequencing approach.

37 *See* National Institute for Clinical Excellence (NICE) website.

Chapter Three

38 *Galanthus caucasicus* is an invalid name but is still sometimes used by those selling this snowdrop.

39 The double snowdrop, now known as *G. nivalis* 'Flore Pleno', was first illustrated by Kychicus in 1703–1705 in the *Duchess of Beaufort's Flowers*, reproduced by Cottesloe, G., Hunt, D. (1983).

40 'Atkinsii' was named by Allen in 1891 saying it was 'second to none in size, form, quality and freedom of growth.' There is possible confusion as to whether the original 'Atkinsii' is available, as my clone does produce deformed flowers on occasional plants.

Chapter Four

41 Bishop, M., Davis, A., Grimshaw, J. (2006).

42 Bishop, M., Davis, A., Grimshaw, J. (2006); Cox, F. (2018); and Kilpatrick, J., Harmer, J. (2018).

43 Bishop, M., Davis, A., Grimshaw, J. (2006); Cox, F. (2018); and Kilpatrick, J., Harmer, J. (2018).

44 Grand Princess Olga Konstantinovna (1851–1936) was a Romanov of the Russian Royal family, who married George I of Greece in St Petersburg in 1867, becoming Queen Olga of Greece.

45 Bishop, M., Davis, A., Grimshaw, J. (2006).

46 Bishop, M., Davis, A., Grimshaw, J. (2006).

47 Bishop, M., Davis, A., Grimshaw, J. (2006).

48 Griffith, M., Yaish, W. F. (2004).
49 Bishop, M., Davis, A., Grimshaw, J. (2006).
50 Bishop, M., Davis, A., Grimshaw, J. (2006).
51 Bishop, M., Davis, A., Grimshaw, J. (2006).

Chapter Five

52 Bishop, M., Davis, A., Grimshaw J. (2006).
53 Cox, F. (2018).
54 Kilpatrick, J., Harmer, J. (2018).
55 Bishop, M., Davis, A., Grimshaw J. (2006).
56 Cox, F. (2018).
57 Kilpatrick, J., Harmer, J. (2018).
58 *See* Stern, F. (1956) p. 70.
59 Bishop, M., Davis, A., Grimshaw J. (2006).
60 Simon Biddulph (2010), personal communication.
61 Bishop, M., Davis, A., Grimshaw J. (2006).
62 Bishop, M., Davis, A., Grimshaw J. (2006).
63 'Kinked' defines a pedicel that has a sharp bend between the pedicel and the ovary, e.g. in 'Galatea'.
64 *See* Davis, A. P. (1999) p. 234.
65 Pratt A. (1873).
66 *See* note 27.
67 *Royal Commission on Historical Monuments, England,* (1939) pp. 100–101.
68 *It was founded in 1298, see Royal Commission on Historical Monuments, England,* (1939), p. 123.
69 See Chapter One 'History of the snowdrop'.

Chapter Six

70 Gerard, J. (1633).
71 Gunther R. T. (1922), *see* p. 311 where 'Snowe Dropps' are listed as growing in 1615, in the garden of Richard Shanne of Yorkshire.
72 Church A. H. (1908).
73 Dodoens, R. (1568).
74 Dodoens', L'Obel's and L'Ecluse's herbals were all published by Plantin in Antwerp, and the same snowdrop woodcut, retained by the publisher, was reused. Gerard's herbal of 1597 reproduces a different snowdrop woodcut, although the later and larger Thomas Johnson's second edition of Gerard in 1633 uses the earlier Plantin image of the snowdrop. Most of Gerard's woodcuts, published in London, made use of the Plantin woodcuts. Indeed, Johnson, in his preface, admits this. He states: 'Now I come to particulars, and first of figures: I have, as I said, made use of those wherewith the Workes of Dodonaeus, Lobel and Clusius were formerly printed…'. Thus the woodcuts of the common snowdrop, *G. nivalis* in Figure 2 (from Gerard,

1633) and Figure 77 (from Dodoens, 1568) are the same, but the caption naming the snowdrop (in Latin) differs. However, a similar Latin caption is in use in Figure 3 (from Gerard,1633) and Figure 79 (from L'Ecluse, 1601) for identical woodcuts of the Crimean snowdrop, *G. plicatus*. See note 8 for further details.

75 L'Obel, M. (1576).

76 L'Ecluse, C. (Clusius) (1583).

77 Gerard, J. (1633).

78 Matthioli, P. (1554).

79 Matthioli, P. (1583).

80 L'Ecluse, C. (Clusius) (1583).

81 L'Ecluse, C. (Clusius) (1601)

82 Brunfels, O. (1536).

83 Fuchs, L. (1542), *see* copy in Magdalen College Library, Oxford.

84 *See* Arber, A. (1938) for the early history of botanical illustration.

85 *See* Blunt, W. (1950) for the history of botanical illustration up to 1950.

86 Dodoens, R. (1586).

87 Passe, C. de (1614).

88 Besler, B. (1613).

89 Parkinson, J. (1629), *see* p. 110 for a description of the common and Crimean snowdrops.

90 Thornton, R. J. (1807); Grigson, G., Buchanan, H., Stern, W.T. (1972).

91 Passe, C. de (1614).

92 Pratt, A. (1873).

93 Hulme F. E. (1875–1900).

94 Sowerby, J. (1790–1814).

95 Curtis, W. (1787–2020).

96 Blunt, W. (1950).

97 Baxter, W. (1834).

98 Clapham, A. R, Tutin, T. G., Warburg, E. F. (1958).

99 Clapham, A. R, Tutin, T. G., Warburg E. F. (1957–1965).

100 Blamey, M., Fitter, R., Fitter, A. (2003).

101 Jacquie Hibbert, personal communication (2018).

102 Jacquie Hibbert, personal communication (2018).

Chapter Seven

103 *See* notes 2 and 3.

Chapter Eight

104 Bishop, M., Davis, A., Grimshaw J. (2006).

105 For further details of these and other living, eminent galanthophiles, see Davis, A. P. (1999); Kilpatrick, J., Harmer, J. (2018); and Cox, F. (2018).

106 *See* note 27.

Glossary

Acetylcholine	A neurotransmitter responsible for conducting electrical impulses across synapses in brain and nerves
Acetylcholinesterase	An enzyme that catalyses the breakdown of acetylcholine
AGM	Award of Garden Merit by RHS
Alzheimer's dementia	A progressive neurodegenerative disease characterized by loss of memory and cognition
Amaryllidaceae	The Amaryllis family in which the snowdrops are classified by taxonomists
Anther	The part of the stamen containing the pollen
Antifreeze proteins	Naturally occurring proteins that protect against freezing
Applanate (vernation)	Leaves lie flat against one another in bud (and at the base of the leaves emerging from the soil)
Bioinformatics	Study of information, often DNA sequence, in biological systems
Botrytis	Fungal pathogens that can kill snowdrops
Bulbous violets	Old name for snowdrops
Byzantine early bulbous violet	Old name for *G. plicatus*
Calligraphy	Beautiful handwriting
Candlemas Bells	Old name for snowdrops
Chromolithography	A process (nineteenth century) for producing multicoloured prints
Clone	Unique isolate perpetuated by vegetative reproduction
Cultivar	Variant within a species selected for cultivation
DNA	Deoxyribonucleic acid, the inheritable compound of most organisms

Double snowdrops	Snowdrops with many small aberrant florets replacing the sexual parts of the flower
Elephant folio	A large size of paper; larger than folio or quarto
Enzymes	Catalysts, usually proteins, that speed up chemical reactions
Explicative (vernation)	Leaf margins folded under in the bud (and at the base of the leaves emerging from the soil) almost touching the back of the leaf
Fair Maid of February	Old name for snowdrops
Filaments	Stalk of the stamens
Flore Pleno	A double flower
Folio	Large paper size used for printing
Galantamine	A naturally occurring toxic compound found in snowdrops, daffodils and other Amaryllidaceae
Galanthophile	A person passionate about snowdrops
Galanthus	Generic name for snowdrops
Genus	The classification hierarchy above that of species
Gerard's herbal	English compendium of useful plants, 1597; first previous use of the word 'snow drop' in Gerard (1633)
Glaucous	A greyish or bluish-grey bloom covering the leaf
Hiemalis	Latin for winter
Hybrid	A plant produced by crossing two different species
Leucojum	Generic name for snowflakes
Linnaeus, Carl	Swedish botanist (1707–1778) who introduced the binomial system of classification
Lodden Lily	Alternative name for Easter snowflake (*L. aestivum*)
Metal plate engraving	Use of a copper plate to prepare prints
Mezzotint	Print from a metal plate engraved to emphasize shadowy effects
Morphology	Appearance of plants used by taxonomists in plant classification
Narcissus violet	Old name for snowdrops

Offset	Naturally occurring new plant, or bulb, easily separated from parent plant
Ovary	Female part of the flower which produces the seeds
Parkinson, John	Author of *Paradisi in sole paradisus terrestris*, or *Garden of all sorts of pleasant flowers* (1629)
Pedicel	The stalk of a single flower
Perianth	The flower – in snowdrops – composed of six segments
Perianth segment	One part of the perianth
pH	Measure of neutrality (pH=7), acidity (pH<7) or alkalinity (pH>7)
Photosynthesis	The process whereby organisms (e.g. plants) use light to synthesize chemicals, usually carbohydrates, from CO_2 and water, thereby generating O_2
Plicate	Upturned leaf margins; more correctly, explicative
Potyvirus	Abbreviation for potato Y virus
Prostrate	On the ground
Proteins	Polymers of amino acids performing many enzymatic and structural functions in cells
Potato Y	A small RNA virus that infects potatoes and snowdrops
RHS	Royal Horticultural Society
Ribosomes	The 'factory' within cells where proteins are made
Ribosomal RNA	RNA found within the ribosome
Ribosomal DNA	DNA coding for ribosomal RNA
RNA	Ribonucleic acid, a nucleic acid with a ribose sugar moiety, e.g. messenger RNA or ribosomal RNA within cells. In some viruses RNA is the inheritable compound
Scape	A leafless stalk arising from the ground
Semi-double snowdrop	Snowdrops with a few small aberrant florets replacing the sexual parts of the flower
Snowflakes	Common name for *Leucojum* species, distinct but related to snowdrops

Spathe	Modified leaves enclosing the flower; each spathe consists of two green spathe valves usually joined by a translucent membrane
Species	The basic classification unit for organisms
Ssp.	Abbreviation for subspecies
Stamen	Male part of flower producing pollen
Stigma	The structure at the tip of the style
Style	The stalk between the ovary and stigma
Subspecies	A distinct group within a species
Supervolute (vernation)	Leaves in bud, and at base of leaves emerging from the soil, wrapped around one another more or less tightly
Taxonomy	Study of classification, e.g. in plants
Tepals	Perianth segments where there is no distinction between sepals and petals
Theophrastus	Greek herbalist of the fourth century BCE
Theophrastus' white violet	Old name for snowdrops or snowflakes
Variant	A plant that differs from the type species, and its normal range of variation, but does not warrant recognition as a different species or subspecies
Vernalis	Latin for spring
Vernation	Leaf arrangement in bud and at base of leaves emerging from the soil
Vignette	Small illustration, borderless, around a capital letter, usually at the beginning of a chapter or book
Virus	A small infectious agent, not free-living, that requires a host to reproduce – not to be confused with a computer virus
Viola alba	Old, ambiguous name for snowdrops, snowflakes and other species
White bulbous violet	Old name for snowdrops
White Ladies	Old name for snowdrops
Woodcut	Print from carved wood

Bibliography: Books, Reports, Web Sites

Arber, A. (1938) *Herbals their Origin and Evolution: A Chapter in the History of Botany, 1470–1670*, 2nd edn. Cambridge University Press.

Baxter, W. (1834–1843) *British Phaenogamous Botany*, 6 vols., Oxford.

Besler, B. (1613) *Hortus Eystettensis,* 3 vols., Nuremberg.

Bishop, M., Davis, A. P., Grimshaw, J. (2006) *Snowdrops – a Monograph of Cultivated Galanthus,* The Griffin Press, Cheltenham, UK.

Blamey, M., Fitter, R., Fitter, A. (2003) *Wild flowers of Britain & Ireland,* Black, London.

Blunt, W. (1950) *The Art of Botanical Illustration,* New Naturalist, vol. 14, Collins, London.

Brunfels, O. (1536) *Herbarium Otto Brunfelsii*, Strasbourg.

Church, A. H. (1908) *Types of Floral Mechanism: A Selection of Diagrams and Descriptions of Common Flowers*, Clarendon Press, Oxford.

Clapham, A. R., Tutin, T. G., Warburg, E. F. (1957–1965) *Flora of the British Isles: Illustrations, Drawings*, parts I–IV, Cambridge University Press.

Clapham, A. R., Tutin, T. G., Warburg, E. F. (1958) *Flora of the British Isles,* Cambridge University Press.

Clusius, *see* L'Ecluse.

Cottesloe, G., Hunt, D. (1983) T*he Duchess of Beaufort's Flowers,* Webb & Bower, Exeter.

Cox, F. (2018) *A Gardener's Guide to Snowdrops*, 2nd edn., Crowood Press, Marlborough.

Curtis, W. (1787–2020) *The Botanical Magazine* or *Flower-Garden Displayed*, London.

Davis, A. P. (1999) *The Genus Galanthus: A 'Botanical Magazine' Monograph*, illustrations by C. King, Timber Press, Portland, Oregon.

Dodoens, R. (1568) *Florum, et coronariarum odoratarumque nonnullarum herbarum historia*, Plantin, Antwerp.

Dodoens, R. (1586) *A New Herbal or History of Plants,* 2nd edn., trans. H. Lyte, London.

Dodonaeus, *see* Dodoens (1568 and 1586).

Fuchs, L. (1542) *De Historia Stirpium*, Basle.

Gerard, J. (1597) *Herball – or Generall Historie of Plantes,* Norton, London.

Gerard, J. (1633) *Herball – or Generall Historie of Plantes,* 2nd edn. T. Johnson, Norton & Whitaker, London.

Griffith, M., Yaish, W. F. (2004) 'Antifreeze proteins in overwintering plants: a tale of two activities', *Trends in Plant Science* 9, 1360–1385.

Grigson, G., Buchanan, H., Stern, W. T. (1972) *Thornton's Temple of Flora with Plates*, Collins, London.

Gunther, R. T. (1922) *Early British Botanists and their Gardens*, University Press, Oxford.

Hulme, F. E. (1875–1900) *Familiar wild flowers,* 5 vols., Cassell, London.

Imhof, D. (2001) 'Return my woodblocks at once: dealings between the Antwerp publisher Balthasar Moretus and the London bookseller Richard Whitaker in the seventeenth century,' in *The Bookshop of the World: The Role of the Low Countries in the Book-trade 1473–1941*, L. Hellinga, A. Duke, J. Harskamp, T. Hermans, E. Paintin (eds.), Goy-Houten, Hes & de Graaf.

Kilpatrick, J., Harmer, J., (2018) *The Galanthophiles: 160 Years of Snowdrop Devotees.* Orphans Publishers, Leominster, Herefordshire.

L'Ecluse, C. (Clusius) (1583) *Rariorum aliquot stirpium per Pannonium, Austrium et vicin*as. Plantin, Antwerp.

L'Ecluse, C. (Clusius) (1601) *Rariorum Plantarum Historia*, Plantin, Antwerp.

L'Obel, M. de (Lobel or Lobelius) (1576) *Plantarum sue stirpium historia*, Plantin, Antwerp.

Lobel, *see* L'Obel (1576).

Matthioli, P. (1554) *Commentarii in sex libros Pedacii Dioscoridis*, Venice.

Matthioli, P. (1583) *Commentarii in sex libros Pedacii Dioscoridis*, Venice.

National Institute of Clinical Excellence (NICE), Donepezil, galantamine, rivastigmine & memantine for the treatment of Alzheimer's disease, www.nice.gov.org.uk/guidance/TA217, updated 20 June 2018.

Parkinson, J. (1629) *Paradisi in sole paradisus terrestris* or *Garden of all sorts of pleasant flowers*, Humfrey Lownes and Robert Young, London.

Passe, C. de (1614) *Hortus Floridus,* Arnhem, Holland.

Pratt, A. (1873) *Flowering Plants, Grasses, Sedges, and Ferns of Great Britain*, 3rd edn., 6 vols., Warne, London.

Ronsted, N., Zubov, D. A., Bruun-Lund, S., Davis, A. P. (2013) 'Snowdrops falling slowly into place: an improved phylogeny for *Galanthus* (Amaryllidaceae)', *Molecular Phylogenetics Evolution*, 69, 205–217.

Royal Commission on Historical Monuments, England (1939) An Inventory of the Historical Monuments in the City of Oxford, His Majesty's Stationary Office, London.

Slade, N. (2014) *The Plant Lover's Guide to Snowdrops*, Timber Press, Portland, Oregon.

Sowerby, J. (1790–1814) *English Botany,* J. Davis, London.

Stern, F. C. (1956) *Snowdrops and Snowflakes,* Royal Horticultural Society, London.

Tabernaemontanus, J. T. (1590) *Eicones Plantarum*, Frankfurt.

Thornton, R. J. (1807) *Temple of Flora*, Thornton, London.

Zubov, D. A., Konka, Y., Davis, A. P. (2019) '*Galanthus bursanus* (Amaryllidaceae): a new species of snowdrop from the Marmara Sea region, NW Turkey', *Kew Bulletin* 74, 18.

Species and Cultivar Index

Numbers in **bold** refer to Figures; cultivars are in inverted commas; species are italicized; *G.* is an abbreviation for *Galanthus*. See Appendix 3, pages 113-114, for an alphabetical list of species and cultivars

GENERAL INDEX

Numbers **in bold** refer to figures

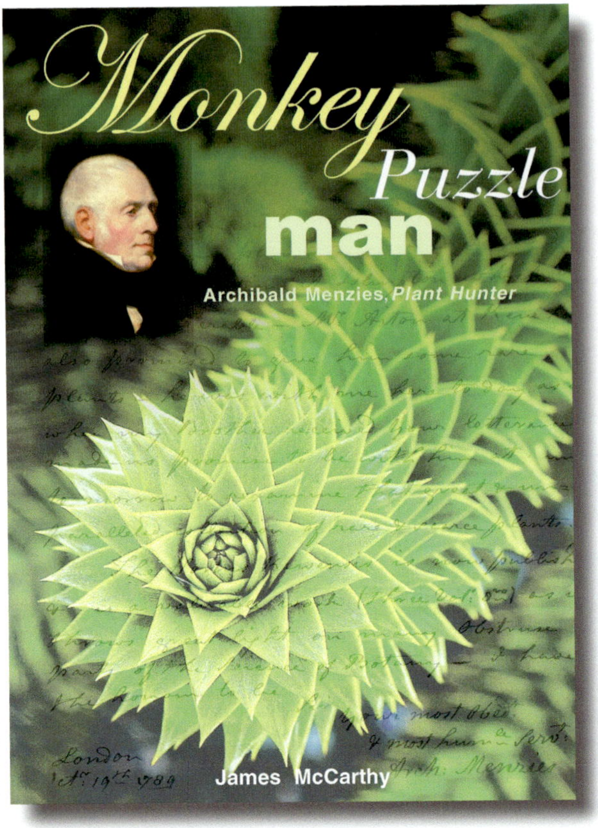

978-1904445-61-6

'... a complete picture of the life of an admirable man with a passion for discovery. And plants.' **Scottish Geographical Journal**

... not just a good read about a plant hunter but also much else about the difficulties of exploration in the second half of the eighteenth century. ... McCarthy has succeeded in putting together a splendid account of a remarkable Scot and enriched the pages with plenty of illustrations in black and white, plus six pages in colour. ... a most professionally written and scholarly work ... this excellent and much recommended book, ...' **BRISC Recorder News**